D1450571

Will I Ever Be the Same Again?

Transforming the Face
of Depression & Anxiety

Carol A. Kivler, MS, CSP

Will I Ever Be the Same Again?

Transforming the Face of Depression & Anxiety

Carol A. Kivler, MS, CSP

Published by:
Three Gem Publishing/Kivler Communications

(609) 882-8988

Cover and Inside Layout: Singles Design

Printed in the United States of America

IBSN: 978-0-9844799-3-1

Dedication

For my mother and father with gratitude and love.

Testimonials for Carol's Mental Health Presentations

"Carol's presentation was the best Grand Rounds we have had at the Cleveland Clinic this year."
Tatiana Falcone, M.D.
Cleveland Clinic

"Your unfailing dedication to breaking down the barriers of stigma related to depression and ECT is exemplary. If only others would have the courage to follow in your footsteps, mental health treatment would no longer be hidden in the shadows. Carol, you are a true gift to humanity. I am personally blessed by your life journey and commitment to improving the quality of life for individuals with psychiatric disabilities and their family members as well as your devotion to bringing the real-world into the academic setting."
Mary D. Moller, DNP, ARNP, APRN, PMHCNS-BC, CPRP, FAAN
Specialty Director, Psychiatric Mental Health Nursing
Yale University School of Nursing

"Both the interns and the more experienced residents were fascinated by Ms. Kivler's talk, and wished for more. She provided living confirmation of many of the things the residents are taught-the effectiveness of ECT, the value of a long term trusting relationship with a

Testimonials for Carol's Mental Health Presentations

psychiatrist, the importance of genuinely listening to the patient, and the impact of ordinary human kindness. The interns could have had no better introduction to the relationship with the patient."

Kimberly R. Best, MD
Albert Einstein Medical Center

"Thank you for your significant contribution to the success of our program. The feedback we received was extremely positive. Most importantly, our guests came away with a call-to-action, many planning to share what they learned and experienced with key stakeholders in their organization. Stories are powerful. They provide context, kindle an emotional fire, and package facts in ways that people will remember and want to share (retell) to others. Thank you for sharing your story, your expertise and your passion for patient education and the power of patient voice in professional education."

Susan R. Grady, MSN, RN-BC
Director, Educational Strategy
and Patient Engagement
MedScape Education

"Carol Kivler's presence at our annual conference elevated the week to "special". She is a top-notch speaker who finds

Testimonials for Carol's Mental Health Presentations

a way to inspire everyone in the audience. But the most remarkable thing about Carol is her generosity of spirit. Coupled with a great sense of humor and love of people, it makes her beloved by those she meets. We are grateful to have met her, and we learned so much. Thank you Carol!"

Wendy Giebink
Executive Director
NAMI South Dakota

"Carol speaks from the heart and shares her personal journey with depression. She brings hope that recovery is possible."

Cathy Epperson
Executive Director
NAMI Kentucky

"Carol Kivler is a gifted speaker with a powerful message that is helping to undo the stigma of mental illness. Her talk is a "must-see" for every medical and mental health professional who thinks they may be sensitive when speaking with patients, but who may be unknowingly perpetuating shame and stigma. Carol's talk will leave you transformed and oriented towards a recovery-mindset."

Corinne Zupko, EdS, LPC, NCC
Adjunct Professor of Counselor Education
The College of New Jersey

Acknowledgments

I would like to acknowledge the many people in my life journey that I consider blessed by their presence. First and foremost, my three amazing children, Kimberly, Russell, and Brandon—their understanding, encouragement, love and support provided the courage I needed to forge ahead with this project.

My two birth sisters, Beverly and Alexis, who I grow closer with each passing year. Mom and Dad continue to send their blessings to all three of us even from heaven.

Lynette Landing, my soul sister, whose creative wordsmithing, unending ideas and fortitude provided a platform to shape this project into reality in record time.

Kathy Dempsey, another soul sister, who believed in my ability way before I believed in myself. Her relentless spirit and passion (and I mean relentless) fueled my own spirit and passion to finally finish this book.

Renee Morelli, one of my best friends, who provided "guiding light" through Reiki from near and far. Her loving spirit knew exactly when I needed a "check-in" call. The card she sent years ago (You Are a Lover of Words, One Day You Will Write a Book) still hangs on my bulletin board in my office.

And finally my utmost gratitude to the many health care professionals at Carrier Clinic and Princeton House whose care I depended on in my darkest moments. Thank you.

Will I Ever Be the Same Again?

Table of Contents

Will I Ever Be the Same Again?

Preface

Twenty years ago, I went through the first of four terrifying acute depressive episodes that took me to my knees and changed my life forever. That may sound very bleak, but it is not meant to. I believe all things happen for a reason and that in every situation, we are presented with choices. We can crumble from the weight of a drastic situation and forever live in the rubble of our life, or we can take what we've learned and rebuild. Sometimes we have to rebuild over and over again. But each time we rebuild, we come back stronger and wiser for it.

My first acute depression was the worst one in that I had no warning. I wasn't prepared for it, nor was my family. The symptoms were strange to me and it seemed to take forever for my doctor to rule out all the things it could be and to arrive at the conclusion that I was clinically depressed. The diagnosis was like a bitter pill. I was caught up in the stigma like the majority of the world, that depression is a sign of weakness or that it belongs to someone who wallows in negativity. That didn't describe me at all. I was happy, active and an inspiration to those in my life, so why in heaven's name was I diagnosed with depression? And to make matters worse, all the medications that were prescribed to me were useless. I was "medication-resistant"; therefore, I sunk deeper and deeper until the depression almost took my life.

Then I was introduced to electroconvulsive therapy (ECT) commonly known as shock treatment. If the stigmas surrounding depression are harsh, the stigmas surrounding ECT are ruthless. The mere name of the treatment conjured up horrible images in my mind and I couldn't imagine undergoing the treatment or letting anyone know I had even considered it. My road to recovery was riddled with obstacles.

I refused the treatment until I reached a point where there were no other options. Without giving ECT a try, I believe I would have landed in a long-term care facility or possibly dead. Within a few treatments there was a noticeable difference in my affect and mood and within a few months I was in recovery. Thankfully, for me, ECT was the "silver bullet" that saved my life and pulled me back into the world of the living – in my case, the world of the thriving. I couldn't believe a treatment with a seemingly bad reputation could be so effective. Over the next ten years, I relapsed into an acute episode three more times. But I was prepared. I knew what worked for me, so I wasted no time in getting ECT treatments.

Between depressive episodes, I am a fully functioning individual who enjoys life to the fullest. I went back to school to get my master's degree, started my own corporate speaking and training company and authored two books. I chose to live in recovery and I've made many lifestyle changes that help me to maintain recovery for long periods of time.

About ten years ago, I felt the urge to share my story with the world. I wanted to help others like me become aware of depression and to overcome the stigma, as well as to accept the diagnosis and commit to recovery. I wanted to help their loved ones to understand them better, and I wanted to help their health care providers to see life through their eyes. But most of all, I wanted to help those who are medication-resistant to consider a viable treatment (ECT) and to see past the myths and the unsavory commentary. The media has portrayed ECT as a barbaric treatment; a treatment only given to "crazy" people in the dark wards of psychiatric hospitals. This life-saving treatment is as far from that reality as it can be. Sadly, quick decisions based on rumors can cause people to shy away from possible breakthroughs – breakthroughs that could potentially save their lives. Too often, we discount a therapy that has a proven high success rate, because of stigma; yet we embrace unproven therapies that have been polished by public-relations experts. That, more than anything, was my motivating factor for writing this book. But it wasn't easy. I have attempted to write this book for ten years. There were times I thought it would never be completed. My journey was difficult, emotionally trying, as well as a strain on so many of my loved ones. Each time I put pen to paper, memories of the most upsetting moments would stop me, and I began to wonder if the book would ever become a reality.

The time finally came. In 2010, I realized that as an established professional speaker, I had the gift of persuasion and influence. There is so much negativity about ECT, that it has become my life purpose to speak to consumers (and their loved ones) who have exhausted other treatment options and have limited or no knowledge of ECT, or have discounted or rejected it because of stigma. It is a phenomenal treatment option that is sadly misunderstood and overlooked. It is not only safe, but used by smart, successful, happy people, not the stereotype we have been left with by misleading movies. My goal is to provide a layperson's perspective on a treatment option that turned my life around. In addition to changing the face of ECT, I also trust that my reader will gain hope through my journey of recovery and through the steps I took to achieve wellness. After ten years, and with the blessings of my wonderful children, this book is finally a reality. My children said, "Mom, if your story can help even one individual achieve recovery, then you have to share it."

This book is divided into three parts. Part I describes my first acute depressive episode and initial ECT treatments. Part II is advice for consumers, their loved ones and health care providers about understanding both depression and ECT, as well as tips to enter into and maintain recovery. Part III is an update concerning my professional/personal life eight years after writing the first edition of this book.

It is my heartfelt desire that you, my reader, will be encouraged and enlightened through my personal journey as well as through the information I have gathered from those I connect with everyday (from other consumers and health care providers). I pray that if you are a consumer you will choose to rebuild your life, no matter how many times you get knocked down, and that you can celebrate a life in courageous recovery.

Part I

MY JOURNEY AND COURAGEOUS RECOVERY THROUGH CLINICAL DEPRESSION

CHAPTER 1

Why Me – Why Not Me?

It was the spring of 1990 when the Beast first reared its ugly head and came barreling through the walls of my world like a wrecking ball. This unwelcome intruder caught me completely off guard allowing no time to prepare myself or my family for what was ahead. The Beast was Clinical Depression and its unannounced invasion changed my life forever.

I was an unlikely candidate for the "Beast" – clinical depression. I led a charmed life. While my marriage was far from perfect, I still counted my blessings. I was happy, healthy, active, and surrounded by a loving family. My husband was an extremely successful attorney and a good provider. I had three terrific children and the ideal career. We owned a large home, beautifully decorated on a gorgeous, well manicured property. With plenty of money in the bank, my cup was definitely overflowing.

Other than a former brief encounter with post-partum depression after the birth of my third child, I had limited awareness of the "whats" and "whys" of depression. As a matter of fact, when I suffered that bout of post-partum, my gynecologist's sure-cure instructions were so nonchalant that depression seemed almost silly to me. He had said, "If you want to get over this depression quickly, just take my advice: Go home, take a warm bath, have a glass of wine and make love to your husband." *Yeah, right! The only one who felt better…was my husband. And the fact is, he was MIA much of the time!*

Luckily within four months, as I got more sleep, the post-partum subsided and the word "depression" was quietly tucked back into a file I mentally labeled "not part of my character"; and I never dealt with it again. That is, until eleven years later.

As a young mom, I was blessed with a life that very few get to enjoy. My husband's extremely successful law firm enabled me to live a life of my choosing. If I wanted to work, I could work. If I wanted to play, I could play. My children were my main priority and my biggest joy was watching them grow and helping them to develop into successful young adults. I chose to spend the majority of my time providing them with an outstanding childhood. And that they received. They grew up with a mother who was not only present before and after school, but also participated in their school activities volunteering time as homeroom mom, and getting involved with the PTA. They never left for school without a full belly and frequently came home to a fresh-baked snack.

Dinner time was family time, where we focused our attention on each other and our meal, not allowing TV, phone calls or other distractions to interfere with quality time. After dinner, we read together or played board games. Our family practices were far from the norm of the typical American household these days, and I took pride in grooming children who had such a high regard for family values that they later established similar practices with their own families. Yes, I adored raising my children and they knew it. When they weren't in school I made sure to broaden their horizons and expose them to all kinds of activities. I ran them around from Scout meetings, to little league, ice hockey, tap dancing, choir lessons and more. They were fortunate to have the opportunity to try different things and to have a live-in 'Taxi-Mom' who carpooled them and their playmates all over God's green earth. I had no complaints – I was grateful for a lifestyle that would allow me to provide that to them.

We were known as regulars at the local library, since that became our once-a-week hangout. I made sure my kids grew up to appreciate that reading today makes for success tomorrow. To this very day, they feel that books are as much a staple to a healthy life as are fruits and vegetables.

Spirituality was always at the center of my family. We attended weekly Church services and sang in the choir and participated in additional ministries. Since my children were blessed to experience a "want for nothing" lifestyle, I made sure they realized the importance of paying it forward. I encouraged them to have an attitude of compassion for others. They often heard me say, "Behind every person is a story, so never sit in judgment." Every year around the holidays, we adopted a family and provided Thanksgiving, Christmas and New Year's Day meals to those less fortunate.

While the majority of my time involved developing my children, I also took time to develop myself by going to school. I had a blast taking classes that were not only enriching but fun: cake decorating, flower arranging, a variety of cooking classes and whatever else piqued my interest. And with a husband involved in politics, I helped out with campaigns, hosted events in our home, and also entertained colleagues and business associates. I volunteered for community efforts like the American Cancer Society.

As my children got older, I decided to re-enter the workforce, teaching business courses part time at a local community college. Prior to starting a family I had received a bachelor's degree in business education and I'd taught both high school and college level classes and even taught in a prison. I absolutely loved teaching, so the idea of getting back into that role was very exciting for me. Needless to say, life was rosy. My personal philosophy was, "Life is something to embrace and enjoy" and that was evident to my family, friends, students and anyone else with whom I connected. That's why it came as a complete surprise when everything began to change.

Out of the blue, my world began to come apart. I can't even pinpoint what started the trend of issues that caught my attention. I can only say, with one thing after another I began facing some sort of blow to my well being, either physical or emotional. At first the changes and challenges were subtle and caused little to no concern, but momentum started to build and I found myself going from one doctor to another to discuss a barrage of symptoms.

Like a chain reaction, lack of sleep eventually became severe insomnia. That triggered nervousness which escalated into major anxiety. Physical symptoms precipitated by anxiety entered the scene causing a loss of appetite, muscle spasms and perpetual headaches. The persistence of all of these symptoms chipped away at my concentration causing a complete lack of confidence and an inferiority complex.

My physical symptoms progressed. I had erratic pains shooting down my arms and pressure in my skull that mimicked the feeling of wearing a helmet. The pain was not only severe, it was constant. It never let up. It eventually wiped out my appetite causing me to lose weight at an alarming rate.

My general practitioner examined me several times as I kept making appointments when new symptoms cropped up. And with each appointment, the doctor would send me for some kind of test: MRI, CAT Scan and the EKG all ruled out several suspected diagnoses. As time crept on and unexplainable symptoms accumulated, my thought process became irrational. Paranoia started to poke and prod at me as I obsessed over my dwindling health, certain I had some kind of terminal illness. I begged my doctor for answers, but after weeks of blood tests and lab work, he still came up empty handed. Finally through the process of elimination, my doctor exhausted all explanations and suggested I see a psychiatrist. *A shrink? Was I going crazy?*

The doctor went on, "I believe you are in a depression." Although his advice seemed illogical to me,

I had no other choice. I certainly didn't want to continue feeling this way, so I went in search of a psychiatrist. *Depression? What do I have to be depressed about? I lead a charmed life.* The shrink I went to see gave a name to the relentless Beast who showed no mercy on me, not even to a person with such an optimistic view of life. That was the day I met my enemy head on – clinical depression.

CHAPTER 2

Where the Heck Is Carol Kivler?

The woman in the mirror staring back at me was barely recognizable. She was pale and drawn with large, dark circles under her eyes. Her previous zest for life had taken what seemed like a permanent leave of absence. *Where is Carol Kivler? What happened to her?* I leaned in a little closer to the mirrored wall in the master bathroom and put a hand on either side of my sunken cheeks wondering if I would ever be the same vibrant, cheerful woman. The one from my former life.

A restful night's sleep was a thing of the past. A mild case of insomnia would have been a welcome change compared to what I was experiencing. Complete sleep deprivation had taken over. No matter how active I was or how much I got done in a day, I just couldn't fall asleep. I felt robbed of the birthright that everyone else in my house got to enjoy, so while they were in a peaceful slumber, I paced the floors of my house, aimlessly wandering from one room into another.

I rubbed my fingers across the deep crevices that recently formed on my forehead, and tried hard to remember what the psychiatrist had explained to me only days before. Our conversation was a blur to my disoriented mind. The appointment with the psychiatrist seemed surreal to me. I never imagined I'd be discussing my mental well being with anyone, let alone a shrink. If feeling like hell the last few months wasn't bad enough, sitting in her office sunk me to a whole new low. *What am I doing here?* There was such a mixture of feelings swirling around my head; relief, denial, confusion, embarrassment. She did her best to make me feel comfortable and respected. We discussed my personal health history, my family's health history, my recent symptoms, and my outlook on life prior to the symptoms, as well as all the tests my doctor had ordered.

She asked me a battery of questions and then turned to my husband to get his perspective on the same questions, all while writing notes on a legal pad. After she finished her fact gathering, she offered up her unequivocal diagnosis. Clinical Depression. My puzzled expression elicited a quick response from her. She must have figured by the look on my face that I equated depression to personal weakness, because she took the ball and ran with it – defining depression, clarifying the different types and explaining how it can affect even those who are happy in life.

She explained that my depression was not brought on by situations or sadness. It was brought on by a chemical imbalance, a disconnect with the neurons in my brain. She talked symptoms, causes, statistics, treatments and side effects. Even though she was making a conscious effort to talk to me in layman's terms, I couldn't keep up. The appointment was a mixture of sheer exhaustion and intense anxiety. As the session continued, my concentration all but diminished. My attention kept drifting, and while I was busy coaxing my focus back on the doctor, I would miss out on full sentences. Too embarrassed to make her repeat herself, I'd just let it go. It was odd – I was aware of the words that came out of her mouth, but they disappeared into thin air before they could penetrate my logical mind. *I'm an intelligent woman, but I can't even follow along.* I felt stupid and useless, barely able to comprehend what the doctor said, yet so desperate to understand. *Where is my head at?* The Beast had imprisoned me in some sort of glass room, where I could see, hear and talk, but could not really engage. The harder I tried to focus, the thicker the glass wall became that separated me from the rest of the world. I glanced over at my husband thankful that he was there to take it all in – to listen attentively to the doctor, to gather up her instructions, and to later translate the information to me. I watched the exchange between him and the doctor and relaxed a little in my chair giving a break to my pounding head.

The Beast was gaining on me, deliberately draining me of the ability to pay attention. With my husband entrenched in conversation with the doctor, I surrendered the task of accumulating facts and instructions about my diagnosis and lapsed into the lull of hope that being diagnosed now provided. *Thank you God, that it's not cancer.* As perplexed as I was about depression and why it decided to knock on my door, I was also relieved that I could finally be treated.

How ironic – to actually *want* a diagnosis. I had never been one to dwell on illness. Quite the opposite, my life had been so full and happy that there was no time for illness and I had a knack for steering clear of it. Yet, over the last several weeks, it came on like a tsunami. *Face it; you are no longer immune to illness.* Carol Kivler, the one who had always preached mind over matter to stay healthy, had actually spent the last several weeks praying that there was something wrong with her. A diagnosis meant treatment and treatment meant a light at the end of the tunnel. *At least I can be treated.*

My comforting lull was being interrupted by a sad realization. The Beast had succeeded in robbing me of yet another virtue I held dear – the ideal that a positive mind guards one's health. Desperate to feel hope, I forced myself to refocus on the realization that yes, I had finally received my diagnosis. *I can get treatment and feel like the old me again.* The Beast released its grip and momentary comfort returned.

I treasured that sense of solace as the psychiatrist concluded our first session, arming us with prescriptions as well as some answers. As we got out of our chairs prepared to leave her cozy office, she said, "I just want to remind you to be patient with this process. We will get you back on track, but remember that it may take six weeks for the drugs to begin to take effect." *Six weeks? Are you kidding me?* My anxiety level soared to new heights. Panic took over and sounded alarms in my head. *How will I survive six more weeks of this hell?* My eyes darted back and forth between the doctor and my husband as I prepared for his objection to her outrageous closing statement. But instead he shook her hand, smiled and escorted me to the car. We continued on to the pharmacy.

Pacing a path between the dining room and living room, I replayed the final moments in the doctor's office and nervously counted days with my fingers. I had been on the antidepressant and anxiety medications for four days. *Only four days?* That meant I still had over five weeks to go. Through the darkness of the night, I shuffled from room to room, consumed with fear. I tried hard to stifle the anxious thoughts by visualizing something peaceful and happy. I squeezed my eyes closed and searched for a single pleasant image in my mind where I could place my focus. The files in my mind contained nothing. I searched more. Each time I would catch a glimpse of something enjoyable, it was instantly replaced with a disturbing image. The one particular image that became burned into my brain was of myself clinging face-first against the inside wall of a large funnel. The gravitational pull was almost too much for me and the only thing that stopped me from being sucked down the hole into the great abyss was the grip I had on the top edge of the funnel. I held on for dear life. *A few more weeks, hang in there for a few more weeks.*

Will I Ever Be the Same Again?

CHAPTER 3

The Oscar for Best Actress

Weeks passed and my health continued to decline. Not only had the medication failed to relieve the depression and anxiety, but I actually felt that they were making me sicker. I would have been willing to pay the price of annoying side effects, like nausea and diarrhea, if the depression had at least lessened, but that wasn't the case. Sleep deprivation was my biggest enemy impairing my ability to think rationally. My patience was wearing thin and I was constantly fixated on the calendar that hung in the kitchen – counting down the days until relief. Although at this point, I had little hope that relief would ever come.

Thankfully my daily routines well rehearsed over the past years rewarded me by becoming second nature. I could move robotically throughout the day getting chores done without a lot of thought or effort. Familiarity with my routines also offered me the added bonus that I could fake the world into believing I was doing better than I really was. My automatic motions in dealing with daily activities masked the fact that I was a complete basket case. If there was an Academy Award for Best Mechanical Actress, I have no doubt the Oscar would have been awarded to Carol Kivler, good wife, mother, sister, daughter, teacher and friend. All while the Beast had me by the throat on the inside, relentlessly tormenting my mind and body. I hid it well. *And the Academy Award goes to…*

I continued to teach, barely able to keep my composure, but intent on hanging on to finish out the semester that was rapidly winding down. *God forbid I lose my job.* My two closest friends urged me to take the rest of the year off, but there was no way I was going to tell the dean at the college what was going on with me. I could fake it through the remaining days…*or could I?*

Every so often, I'd look up from my desk to catch the odd expressions of my students before they would quickly look away from me. *You can't fool them anymore, they are on to you.* I began to unravel realizing my performance was no longer working. The vibrant woman, who stood at the front of their class earlier in the semester, was now a skeleton of herself. *They know what a fake you are.* No drive, no enthusiasm, and filled with fear. I called my brother-in-law and asked him for help in grading the final exams I was ready to administer.

I was anxious to finish out the semester. Pretending to be a professional was becoming way too difficult, not to mention the drive to and from work. My husband urged me to stop driving after having followed me home one day. "You were all over the road. You are not safe to drive anymore." I agreed to let him drive me around until the medication would kick in and I could get some sleep.

When I wasn't teaching or tending to my own kids, I stood inside my living room, staring out of the window for hours. It was spring time, the most beautiful time of the year, but I couldn't see the sunshine. I didn't notice the baby robins or the squirrels that scampered playfully across the front lawn. I couldn't appreciate the well landscaped yard with the gorgeous shrubs and trees, and the flowers that blossomed right in front of me. I could only see me, hanging by my fingertips, to the top edge of a funnel, fighting the almighty force that tried to pull me down through the hole. And when the image of the funnel finally faded, another disturbing image was waiting there to replace it. I was a bag lady, living on the street. I wore tattered clothes and carried the only few belongings I had. No money, no food, no shelter and no family. Everything was lost. The image was so real it made me shutter. *Hopeless.*

There was a red circular patch of skin on my forehead where it rested against the glass pane and the air exiting my nostrils fogged the window. I held up an exhausted fist and rubbed a clear spot, pushing the moisture out of the way and regaining my view out the window. The moments spent by the window seemed to fuel the Beast more than any other. I could sense the Beast drinking in those moments, becoming bigger and stronger and then turning on me, eager to wreak havoc on my mind. I stared out the window picking apart our property, wondering when the cars would fall apart, and agonizing over our unavoidable financial destitution. The house needed maintenance and upkeep. The paint on the walls was dingy and unappealing. *Who will want to buy this mess of a house when we can no longer afford to keep it?*

There was a shortage of food in the pantry and the refrigerator, so I began to ration meals, giving up my portion entirely to ensure there was enough for the children. My husband tried to reason with me constantly, telling me that I was out of touch with reality and that we were doing just fine and had plenty of food and money. He tried to convince me that I wasn't seeing things clearly because of my state of mind. I scoffed at him and told him to get out of denial. *Why is he lying to me?*

Night after night I wore a beaten path throughout my home, slowly pacing from room to room like a security guard on duty. There was no point in lying down as the anxiety worsened once my head hit the pillow. The chilling images of me living on the streets or dangling from the funnel's edge would return. I'd had enough of those tormenting images all day. Pacing the house seemed to relieve it. Sometimes I would count my foot steps to keep my mind busy.

A month had now passed since I first saw the psychiatrist and started on the medication. No relief. I was far worse off. *Kiss the good life goodbye, you are losing everything.* I mentally chronicled the negative events of the past month. Very few hours of sleep, depression has turned to despair, anxiety is constant, no longer able to drive…have no desire to live. *No desire to live. No desire to live. I want to die.*

It was no secret that I felt this way, but I hadn't had the courage to even admit it to myself, until that moment. *I want to die.* Acknowledging the reality of this thought sent chills down my spine and I started to gag uncontrollably. I ran into the powder room where no one could hear me and I hung my head over the toilet as the dry heaves came on like contractions.

My stupid body, the area of my brain that controls vomiting wasn't aware that there was no food in my stomach and so it kept trying to make me vomit. After several minutes of dry heaving, I panted from exhaustion and pain. Still hanging over the toilet, my eyes watering from gagging, the heaves started to subside giving me the ability to finally say it out loud. *I can't take this anymore. I want to die.*

I watched myself let go of the top edge of the funnel. With no more strength to hold on, my hands gave up their grip and I swirled round and round, lower and lower, slithering slowly and completely down the hole. The Beast raised its arms, stomped its feet and shouted out a victory cry. A white flag waved in the distance. It was me holding it. The Beast bellowed with joy. I left the white flag whipping in the wind and I went to my bedroom. I knew what I had to do.

CHAPTER 4
I Surrender, You Win

There is a peace in letting go. Maybe it's the relief of no longer having to fight the inevitable, of no longer struggling to keep control, of no longer trying to stop the ceiling from caving in. The act of holding the ceiling up for so long is so exhausting and painful that letting it quickly crush me and leave me for dead was an almost soothing concept. I was actually on a high thinking about it. No more worry, no more pain, no more sleepless nights. *I surrender, you win, and I feel at peace.*

It was a glorious day. I stood in the meadow under the warm sun. Birds were chirping and tiny butterflies in different colors added specks of color to the blue sky. I was wearing a peach silk blouse with ruffles and a mocha skirt. I looked like a million bucks. A gentle breeze made my hair bloom out from under my collar. I felt light and beautiful and I spun around drinking in the warmth of the day. I inhaled long and slowly enjoying the feeling of relaxation, the feeling of a pain-free body, and a mind void of all stress. It had been a long time since I felt this wonderful and I wanted to enjoy every second of it. *I am free.* I danced around as if I were ten years old.

The sky darkened. *A storm is coming.* Heavy winds pushed the calm away and the temperature began to drop. Within seconds, thick dark clouds hovered overhead and the sun vanished behind a wall of black. I shivered and struggled to keep my footing. The wind wildly whipped hair into my eyes. The sunny meadow was gone and I stood at the edge of a dark alley that divided a busy city block. Cars raced by beeping their horns. I felt the presence of others and suddenly realized that my children were there with me. Frantically trying to protect them from the dangerous traffic, we darted behind the smelly garbage that was piled as high as I am tall. My clothes were tattered and dirty and my children's faces were covered with grime. We had no idea where to go.

Sitting on the edge of my bed, I realized this vivid hallucination mimicked a nightmare. *Horribly unfair.* I had avoided coming to bed for weeks now since it was a place I despised, a place where the hauntings of depression swirled around my brain the moment my head hit the pillow. Tonight, like many other nights, I had no intention of lying down or sleeping and yet the nightmare I would expect to dodge through being awake, found me anyway. Found me sitting on the edge of my bed. Apparently, the Beast wasn't ready to rest either. It was sending me a message far worse than anything I could imagine. The Beast was not going to settle with just taking me. It wanted my family too.

I glanced at all the family portraits on the walls. The five of us decked out in festive ensembles posed in front of an elegant Christmas tree. A new portrait hung depicting each year, ever since my youngest was born. I hadn't even noticed the portraits in the last week, not since the night my parents visited and pushed the portraits in my face, saying things like, "You've got to snap out of this mood Carol. If not for you, do it for your kids. You are falling apart."

I know they were grappling for something to bring me back to the living. I'm sure it was hard for them to watch my mood rapidly deteriorate. But I couldn't get them to understand that I was empty. I had no feelings for anything! Not myself, not them, not my husband, not my kids. Completely void of feeling anything – anything but fear.

Now as I looked at the portraits, I felt sick to my stomach. *Who will take care of my children? They can't survive without me.* A large knot gripped my stomach. *No one could ever love them like I do. No one! There won't be anyone to help them with homework. No one to take care of them if they get sick.* I could barely breathe to think of them living a life without me. Thoughts of their future sadness and pain made the knot tighten and I almost gagged again. *No one to keep them clean and fed. No one to make sure they stay active and happy. I can't leave them. I have to take them with me.*

I sat back down on the edge of the bed and waited for my husband to wake up. The sun was almost ready to rise. It wouldn't be long now.

"Good morning sweetheart, Happy Mother's Day," my husband mumbled through a yawn while he rubbed the sleep from his eyes. *This is Mother's Day?* How clever of the Beast. A day usually spent with my beloved children enjoying each others' presence. How devastating to think that this was the day I planned to end it all.

"Please, I can't go on like this for another day, you

and the children must come with me," I pleaded. "Come with you where? What are you talking about?" he asked as he sat up in bed looking confused. "No one can love you and the children as much as I do – please, please, please listen to me!"

It took him a minute to register what I was suggesting. He got out of bed and quickly started getting dressed. His sleepy face became somber and he was fully alert. He told me to put on my sneakers. "Let's go for a walk."

He was acutely aware of the fact that my mind had crossed over to the abyss of psychosis with thoughts of not only ending my life but his and the lives of the children as well. He was adamant about getting us both out of the house, not taking any chances that one of our children would overhear our conversation. A conversation that was irrational to the sane mind. Once we were outside I told him my plan.

After our walk, my husband sat me down in the living room and went looking for the children. They prepared an orange juice toast in champagne glasses. He and my three children raised their glasses and wished me a Happy Mother's Day. And then my husband turned to the kids and said, "Mommy is very sick and she is going to the hospital tomorrow so she can get better."

He explained in brief terms that I was going through a depression and that it had nothing to do with them and that the hospital was the best place for me at this point. Then he made them promise him, one at a time that no one would get in the car with me.

CHAPTER 5

My Life in Lockdown

Everything was gray. The walls of the hospital – gray.
The big metal door that kept me imprisoned here – gray.
The faces of all the crazies vacationing here – gray. Even
the scrubs that the entire hospital staff sported – gray.
Couldn't even one nurse find it in their heart to wear a
Winnie the Pooh print?

The lockdown ward had been my home for a couple
weeks now. I wouldn't have been anymore surprised to
find out I was on another planet. Life here was odd to
say the least. One thing that stood out for me was how
every patient seemed to do the same psychiatric
hospital shuffle. Upon checking in, we all lost our ability
to walk normally. Feet never really left the ground as we
slowly scuffed our way through the halls of the ward.
Was it depression or the medication cocktails?

Memories of elementary school resurfaced every so
often, as my fellow patients and I were lined up like sheep
and herded from one activity to the next. "Single file
everyone, and please follow me," a nurse would lead us
into a large room for group therapy or music therapy or
art therapy. "Please line up for medication", and we were
ushered to the drug window where we were handed our
individually prescribed concoction of pills in a tiny paper

cup along with a cup of water. We obediently swallowed our pills and allowed hospital staff to inspect our mouths to prove the meds were consumed. *I made award winning crab puffs a few months ago when my husband and I hosted a dinner for some long-term clients, and now here I am, sticking my tongue out at a nurse to prove I'm not stashing pills under it.*

Although I was never hungry, meal time at least offered a little color to this otherwise gray place. Pushing plastic trays across a metal counter, I made food selections and waited for a staff member to measure my food before I ate it. *How much damage can I do with a plastic knife?* I knew I was on suicidal watch 24/7, so I did my best to put on a façade that appeared to want to live. In the meantime, I was obsessed with suicidal plans. *Can I break that picture frame and slash my artery? Can I use that trash can liner to suffocate myself?*

When I first checked in, they went through my belongings with a fine-tooth comb, removing any sharp objects like tweezers and cuticle scissors or make-up containers that had mirrors that could be broken into shards as weapons. They even took the shoe laces out of my sneakers. That really limited my ability to do myself in. *What do they think I'll do – hang myself with my shoelaces?*

My room had two twin beds, two closets and a small bathroom. There was one window that looked out to a large tree. The first time I stood by the window a thought occurred to me that gave me chills. There were times in my life where the stress level would get so high that I would jokingly tell loved ones, "When they lock me away someday, make sure the room has a window that overlooks a tree, so I can rock." *Had I manifested this whole nightmarish situation with my stupid joke?*

My parents had temporarily moved into my home to take care of the kids when I was admitted here. Almost every day, someone from my family would visit me and try to figure out what happened to me or give me some reason I needed to get better. Mom and Dad frantically questioned my psychiatrist about their parenting practices and if they caused my illness. My sisters sat with me one at a time and urged me to stop withholding the truth and confide in them. Had I committed some kind of crime? Was I having an affair? Was there some dark secret I was keeping from them that had led to this unfortunate situation? And all of them would bring pictures of my kids in an effort to wake me up from this disconnect. *How can I make them understand? I can't control this Beast!* I did my best to act "normal" when family members were around. But I'd lost the sense of what "normal" was, especially hanging around the community room where some patients sat facing the gray walls mumbling to themselves. The "no visitors allowed" hours of the day became the easiest for me to deal with as I lulled into the land of the lost.

The "Love Boat" offered a number of activities for us crazy cruisers to choose from. Each day we could take yoga, dance class, assertiveness training, or horticulture. We could exercise, meditate, make crafts, or attend some kind of religious ceremony. A hospital worker lowered the volume on the TV for a moment to announce that a priest was about to begin mass in the "Big Room." I immediately stopped what I was doing to attend mass. The next day, the hospital worker announced that a rabbi was about to begin services. I quickly headed to the Big Room to attend. The next day, I attended the Protestant service with the minister…and finally the perplexed looking staff member came up to me and said, "Carol, what religion are you?" It didn't matter. All I knew was during that blissful hour of God's time, I could escape the Beast.

Twenty five days into my stay, I showed no signs of progress. No response to the ever changing combination of drugs, and still wishing I was dead, the psychiatrist sat down with my husband and I and recommended ECT (electroconvulsive therapy). *Shock therapy? Are you kidding me? No way!*

I couldn't believe it had come to this! The doctor was suggesting something so barbaric, something only the craziest and most unstable of people would undergo. Not me! No matter what the doctor said about it, I could only envision the catatonic characters in the movie "One Flew Over the Cukoo's Nest" and I shook my head no, not even willing to listen to his reasoning. When the appointment concluded, my husband said "Why wouldn't you even listen to the doctor? It sounds to me like…"

I cut him off cold, "People who get that treatment end up staring into space forever! They sit and rock and drool!"

"But Carol," he urged "nothing has helped you so far, why won't you at least consider it?"

"Why don't YOU just get zapped and tell me how YOU like it!" I snapped back and then turned my back on him and walked towards my room.

Over the next few days, the staff labeled me "unwilling to comply" but continued to try to sell me on the shock treatment. They said that because my depression hadn't budged, it was the next best option. My parents also jumped on the band wagon. With everyone hounding me, I agreed to at least watch a film about the process. But in my paranoid state of mind, the film only frightened me, pushing the idea further away from me. The only option to free me from the Beast was this brutal form of treatment. My psychosis worsened and my suicidal ideation was at an all time high as I continually looked for a way out of this misery.

My doctor and family members must have read my mind because they began a relentless campaign to convince me to receive shock therapy. They wouldn't ease up until I finally surrendered. "Okay I'll do it. I'm sick and tired of being bullied!" Another family meeting was held to describe the procedure and have me sign the medical waiver. I felt like I was signing away all control of my life. *I'd rather die now than live the rest of my life in some twilight zone just to make everyone else happy.* My husband let out a sigh of relief as I signed the paper agreeing to begin treatment the very next day. The meeting adjourned and everyone went their separate ways satisfied with their accomplishment. I lay in bed facing another evening of insomnia. This one, worse than any other.

My husband showed up the following day, earlier

than usual. He was bubbling over with excitement to hear the results of my first jolt-to-the-brain experience. *He's not going to like what he hears.* He approached the chair where I sat facing the window and handed me a small bunch of flowers wrapped in cellophane. "For you honey." Then he touched my shoulder and said "How did it go today?"

"I passed on it." I continued to stare out the window and laid the flowers down on the sill in front of me.

"What? What do you mean?" Through the reflection in the glass, I could see his shoulders droop. "I was there when you signed the medical release last night."

"I couldn't go through with it! I couldn't relax last night knowing I was going to get electrocuted today so I went to the nurse's station and had them pull my form. I just couldn't do it!"

"You changed your mind and didn't discuss it with me?" his tone obviously annoyed. "Why are you refusing to comply?" He leaned on the door jam suddenly looking exhausted.

My jaw tightened. "Look, this is MY life! And it's no small decision! It's not like I'm trying to decide which handbag to purchase! This is a big deal! It affects my future, my family, my career…I don't expect you to understand." I stopped talking when I noticed his whole disposition changed before my eyes. Throughout this whole ordeal, I had yet to see my husband look aggravated with me. Concerned, confused, sad at times, but never aggravated. That changed tonight. He stared right at me, yet his thoughts were a million miles away.

His lips parted as if ready to say something but nothing came out. Another minute went by without a word and then he stepped towards me abruptly, leaned over to kiss my cheek and told me he had to go take care of some things and he was out the door. *He looks defeated.*

My heart sunk. I hated disappointing anyone, but I was scared to death! Still sitting in the chair in front of the window, I let out a desperate sigh and dropped my head back, gazing into space. *God please help me! I don't know what to do!*

Will I Ever Be the Same Again?

CHAPTER 6

It's My Secret –
No One Has to Know

During dinner, one of the nurses, Diana, approached me as I was finishing up my meal. She asked if we could talk in private. I threw away my garbage and placed my plastic tray with the others on the dirty dish cart, and then followed Diana down the hall and into a small lounge near the nurse's station where we sat together on a brown leather sofa.

I didn't know what this was about, but I instantly felt comfortable around Diana. She had a tiny build and curly auburn hair and her demeanor was gentle. Even before she got to the point of this face-to-face, I could tell she really cared about me. I don't know if it was the tone of her voice, or the look in her eyes, but I knew right away, she was my ally. *I trust her.* This was unusual for me as most of the staff intimidated me. I spent the first couple weeks tensing up each time a hospital worker came near me, fearful of their motive. *What if they take advantage of me in my vulnerable state? Who will protect me?*

"Carol," Diana said, "In all the years I've worked here, I have never seen a more dedicated family. They love you so much and want to see you get well. We want to see you get well too. But Carol, you're no better than the day you arrived here. You aren't responding to any of the medications you've taken, and I believe ECT may hold the key to getting you back to your old self again." She paused and then touched my hand, "You have to do this for them Carol – for your family. Your husband wants his wife back and your children want their mother back." She looked at me for some kind of response, but I just sat there quietly. "I promise you can trust me. Talk to me and tell me why you are so afraid of the ECT, and I will do my best to ease your mind."

Her calm and caring air soothed my spirit and enabled me to talk openly. I shook my head in a way to let her know I was listening as I attempted to organize my thoughts and said, "To be honest, it isn't the actual treatment that scares me so much…it's the idea of everyone knowing! God…what will they think? What will they say?"

"But Carol, your husband, your parents…your sisters; they're all on board with the idea…"

I waved my hand back and forth in front of her, "No Diana, you don't understand. What will my colleagues say? What will the dean at the college say? And what about the neighbors? Will they ever let their children come over to my house to play with my children again? What will they think of me?"

The corners of her mouth turned up and a small smile replaced the previous look of concern on Diana's face. She tipped her chin down slightly and took her voice down to a whisper. "But Carol, they don't have to know! Don't you see? This can be your secret! No one needs to know!"

No one needs to know. She's right! No one needs to know, and it can be my secret! For the first time in a long time, I think I actually smiled. A tiny smile, but a smile none the less. *A turning point.*

The next day, I waited for someone to come get me for my first shock treatment. I tried hard not to think about what I was ready to undergo. I focused on the large tree outside my window and wondered how many years it stood there looking on at the various consumers that stayed in this very same room. Did it have any idea what we were going through? Why we were even here? The bright green leaves that dangled from the branches suddenly danced back and forth from a random gush of wind, as if to wave at me. *Are you acknowledging my thoughts? Are you commiserating with me because you feel the same sadness I do? Or are you mocking me?*

A familiar voice entered my room. I turned around and exhaled a breath I had held for God only knows how long. *Thank goodness.* I was so relieved to see my ally was on duty today. Compassionate, smiling Diana. "I'm so proud of you Carol. You made the right decision," she said.

"I'm glad you're here."

"I'll be with you for the whole procedure. As a matter of fact, I promise mine is the last face you'll see before you are put to sleep and the first face you'll see when you awake after the treatment." *Put to sleep...now there's a perk I hadn't thought of – I'll finally get some sleep.*

"Okay, they are ready for us. Let's head downstairs to the ECT Suite," she said and pointed in the direction we should head. *Suite? Should I expect five-star service and a mint on my pillow?* An interesting choice of words, although I guess it was better than calling it the ECT Chamber. A few medical professionals were there waiting for me and kindly introduced themselves to me and then prepared me for the treatment.

Behind a curtain, I removed my mismatched clothes and put on a hospital gown that tied in the front. I climbed up on the table with the crisp white sheet spread across and lay facing up as the pros began connecting all kinds of things to me. They took my pulse and my temperature and wrapped a blood pressure cuff around the upper part of my left arm. An IV needle pierced the bulging vein in my right arm, and was taped into place so it wouldn't move. I stared at the ceiling tiles above me. They explained what they would do once I fell asleep, like putting a bite-block in my mouth and attaching probes to my head. And then a tall slim young man with light blue eyes and a chiseled face stood at the head of the table I was lying on. He bent over me slightly making his face enter my upside down view and he smiled and told me to relax and enjoy the ride. "You will start to feel sleepy now Carol." Immediately, I could sense the anesthesia filtering into my system slowly and wonderfully – a tickling sensation from the inside out. *How pleasant is this.* An interesting echo filled my head replacing all my cares and anxiety, and I floated through space, light as a feather. As promised, Diana stood by my side and looked into my eyes as they fought to stay open. "Relax Carol, I'll see you shortly." She squeezed my hand as I drifted peacefully... peacefully asleep.

CHAPTER 7
Return to the Living

Five days and three treatments had past since I had first visited the "Suite." I began to look forward to the short period of sleep that each treatment provided. It didn't matter that it was induced sleep – at least it was sleep. *Sleep, glorious sleep.* The headaches that resulted from the routine treatments were not as bad as I had anticipated, so I was thankful for that. I did notice my short term memory was affected and sometimes the days would run together and I would lose all track of time or forget something someone said. But then again, severe depression had done its best to destroy my mental faculties for months now, so these "side-effects" were nothing to fret over. My husband came for his daily visit shortly after I finished with my third treatment. As soon as we made eye contact, his eyes welled up with tears and he started to cry. "Carol," his voice cracked, "I can see a difference! I see a sign of life in your face again!" Even though I hadn't felt much of a difference, I could tell by his reaction that he saw a real change and that was encouraging to me.

Over the next few weeks, my ECT treatments continued three times per week. With each treatment, I could feel myself slowly but steadily being released from the grips of the Beast. After months of sleep deprivation, the greatest gift was that of progressively gaining more hours of sleep each night. With more rest, my anxiety decreased and my hallucinations and thoughts of suicide dissipated. The darkness began to lift.

During a music therapy class one day, the therapist began to play the piano and asked if anyone in the room would like her to play a particular song. I thought about a tune my daughter and I use to sing from the movie Ice Castles.

"Do you know the song I'm talking about?" I asked the therapist.

"Yes I do!" she said and immediately began playing it.

Hearing the song did something to me that I wasn't expecting. Tears instantly flooded my eyes, spilling down over my cheeks and splashing on the table in front of me. The first tears I'd cried since the Beast took them away months ago. My emotions had been buried in some deep dark place for so long now that I'd forgotten how it felt to…feel. And now my long lost spirit that had been left for dead finally managed to get free and follow a tiny spark of light up to the surface. The tears kept coming. Tears of relief, sorrow, disappointment and loneliness and even tears of joy for the sake of feeling again. *There is hope.*

After 38 days in the hospital, I was released, but continued with the ECT treatments on an outpatient basis. I was exhausted but functioning, okay for someone who had just spent over a month in the hospital and had received over a dozen shock treatments. I was still far from feeling like my old self, but at least I had a morsel of faith that I was on the road to recovery. And I found something that I could hold on to – a hush-hush, misunderstood and often rejected form of treatment eventually gave me back my life.

My reentry into the world of the living was slow and subtle. I cautiously collected bits and pieces of my old self, completely unaware that I was getting better until someone would point something out. My children were especially good at that. I asked my daughter to plug in my curling iron one day, so I could set my hair before going to church. She turned to me with tears in her eyes and said, "Mom, you are coming out of the depression; you haven't combed your hair in weeks and now you want to set it!" I'd catch her smiling every so often, "What are you thinking about sweetie?" I would ask, and she'd tell me how good it was to see me wearing jewelry again, or putting on lipstick, or being the fashion conscious mom from before. Or my middle son who would say "Mom, you must be getting better 'cause you're finally making sense again." The simplest things were constant indications that I was coming back to me. One day I found myself sitting alone, taking in all my surroundings. *This house is so beautiful! I am really blessed! And it hit me – the realization that Carol Kivler was back.*

I'd like to say that I never had another encounter with the Beast, but that isn't the case. Three more over-whelming episodes of clinical depression encroached on my happy home in the next nine years. But ECT became my silver-bullet, hitting the Beast right between the eyes and keeping it at bay, while quickly returning me to normal again. In between depressive episodes, I was a productive member of society, going back to school for my master's degree, and building my business. Without ECT, I'm certain that would not be the case. My biggest obstacle concerning recovery became accepting ECT as a viable treatment. But then some of the biggest heroes and heroines in history have been given a bum rap. Ignorance can cost us precious time, not to mention a lot of pain and suffering and maybe even our lives. After being rescued four different times, I vowed to change the world's perception of my hero. Shock therapy not only kept my depression in check, it gave me the ability to reconnect and fully appreciate all the wonders in life, especially my beautiful children. Without ECT, I may very well have missed out on one of the greatest joys in my life – eventually becoming "Grammy."

Recovery: More Than a Possibility, It's a Probability

In the past, many people with psychiatric diagnoses were told straight out that there really wasn't any hope that they would be able to reclaim a full or productive life. And each time I speak to an audience about "living in recovery" they are astonished to learn that recovery is possible from clinical depression. They are literally awed to learn that the cheerful, successful, well "put-together" woman standing before them was in a psychotic state twenty years earlier. They are even more surprised to learn that between depressive episodes I went back to school, completed my master's degree, left my job teaching at the college and opened my own training company. Yes, recovery is not only possible, it is probable.

When I was first diagnosed with clinical depression, I asked myself, "Why me?" In trying to understand my new diagnosis, I researched information and discovered how prevalent the disease is, and my question then became "Why not me?"

Years later, when I began to speak openly about my experiences of living with clinical depression and undergoing shock treatments, I realized I was far from alone in my old style of thinking. With increased knowledge, my newly formed perception concerning clinical depression crumbled the wall of ignorance that I once knew. The majority of the general population is ignorant when it comes to depression and ECT. Lack of knowledge spawns ignorance. Ignorance generates fear. And fear leads to stereotyping and stigma.

The word "stigma" is derived from Latin for a tattoo indicating slave or criminal status. Many popular dictionaries define stigma as a mark of infamy, disgrace or reproach. The current stigmas surrounding depression are so harsh that it is estimated that only about half of those struggling with depression seek treatment. Have they bought into the stigma? Do they fear rejection from others?

While it seems that the overall understanding of clinical depression has progressed over the last twenty years, I believe there is still a long way to go.

My goal in the second half of this book is to create an awareness of a common yet misunderstood illness – clinical depression. I also hope to expose the most common stigma attached to both clinical depression and ECT. Through my own experience as well as the experiences of others with whom I have spoken I hope to offer tips to enrich and enhance the lives of the consumers, their loved ones and the health care providers who all have an association with clinical depression. It is my hope that imparting more knowledge will lead to many more courageous survivors.

Part II

VALUABLE TIDBITS FOR HEALTH CARE PROFESSIONALS, CONSUMERS AND THEIR LOVED ONES

Will I Ever Be the Same Again?

CHAPTER 8

Changing the Face of Clinical Depression

Imagine meeting someone at work, at the gym or at some social function and finding out they have clinical depression. What would your immediate reaction be? Would you think of them as negative minded? Selfish? Weak? Unintelligent? Crying out for attention? Believe it or not, these are all common reactions and misconceptions. Due to a lack of knowledge, people often say or think the following things about people who are depressed:

He's not depressed, he's just lazy!

It's no wonder she's depressed, she's always wallowing in self-pity.

If he would stop focusing on the negative all the time, he might not be depressed!

These ideas have been ingrained in us so strongly that many people who encounter depression deny themselves treatment because they are too busy judging themselves when they can't pull through the disease alone. Those who are in the midst of depression often find themselves thinking:

I am a complete failure.

There's no way I will go for treatment and let others think I'm weak!

God must be punishing me.

Major depression is not an attitude. It is not a personality dysfunction. It is not a flaw in character. It is not laziness or a call for attention. It is not hurt feelings or a reaction to a bump in the road. It is not contagious. Depression is not something that can be brought on or fought off by self-will. Depression is not something to be ashamed of. And most importantly, it is not something that should be ignored. Left untreated, serious depression can be life-crippling and even lead to death (by suicide).

No one wants to be depressed. So what is depression? Depression is real. Clinical depression is an illness and can affect anyone at anytime just like any other illness: diabetes, high blood pressure, asthma, heart disease, cancer, etc. Depression is an illness of the mind just like diabetes is an illness of the pancreas. Have you ever told a diabetic to "snap out of it"? Probably not, yet why is it that the average person is much less compassionate and much more critical when a diagnosis falls under the umbrella of "mental illness"? With little to no awareness about the facts concerning clinical depression, those who have the illness are unlikely to seek help, and those who know someone with the illness may make incorrect assumptions and act in an unsupportive way.

Research shows that images of the brain appear different in those with depression than from those who are not depressed. In non-depressed people, brain areas that regulate mood, thinking, appetite and sleep appear to function normally, whereas in a depressed person there is abnormal activity shown in the brain imaging. Depression is an illness that affects the physical body, not just the emotions.

While there are many types of depression, my goal is to help you distinguish between **situational depression and clinical depression**. Situational depression is typically caused by some sort of change, loss, or difficulty in one's life. Therefore, the depression is directly related to the situation that triggered it. A severed relationship by separation or death, the loss of a job or hobby, a forced relocation, a global catastrophe or having witnessed a tragedy are just a few examples of situations that can trigger depression. In most cases, situational depression is temporary and the passing of time will alleviate the sadness, grief, insomnia, or other symptoms associated with the depression.

Clinical depression is a mental illness that is distinguishable from feeling sadness or grief because it lasts for more than a couple of weeks or months. While the illness may be triggered by a situation like death, loss or difficulty, the most important thing to remember is that clinical depression is not temporary nor will the passing of time alleviate the symptoms. Clinical depression is an illness that requires treatment and lifestyle changes. It is a severe type of depression (also called major depression) that causes a loss of interest in usual activities and challenges your ability to perform your daily routine. It affects any and all races, ages, ethnic and religious backgrounds and socio-economic factors.

Clinical depression shows up as abnormalities in the chemical make-up or neurotransmitters of the brain. These abnormalities are biological and not caused by situations or anything that you did. The neurotransmitters are said to be out of balance.

To understand more about depression and the symptoms associated with it, I have included the following self-assessment. Check the box in front of any of the statements with which you agree:

❑ I am sad almost all of the time.
❑ I have difficulty finding the energy to do even the simplest things.
❑ I have lost interest in most of the things I found enjoyable.
❑ I just want to sleep all the time and have difficulty getting out of bed to face the day.
❑ I am restless and find it difficult to sleep.
❑ I have lost my desire to eat – I have no appetite.
❑ I have lost interest in sexual intimacy.
❑ I am not able to focus or concentrate like in the past.
❑ I forget things and find it difficult to make even simple decisions.
❑ I am irritable and frustrated with everyone and everything.

- ❑ I have no desire to socialize and I avoid social functions.
- ❑ I don't feel up to talking to people.
- ❑ I feel achy and have physical pains that won't go away.
- ❑ I have constant anxiety and fear, but I can't pinpoint why.
- ❑ Nothing makes me happy and I feel like there isn't much point in living.
- ❑ I worry about things that rarely bothered me before.
- ❑ I feel bad about myself and don't like what I see in the mirror.
- ❑ I find myself thinking about death a lot and wishing I could end my sadness.
- ❑ I sometimes think about how I might kill myself.

If you checked several of the items you may have depression. Don't wait. Make an appointment with your doctor to discuss the things you have checked in the list. You deserve to feel better. So take the first step.

Will I Ever Be the Same Again?

CHAPTER 9

Demystifying ECT (Electroconvulsive Therapy)

Electroconvulsive therapy is a customary psychiatric procedure used to treat severe major depression that has not responded to other treatments. ECT uses a therapeutic dose of electricity to induce a seizure to the brain of an anesthetized patient. My depression was so severe that if it weren't for ECT, I'm quite certain I would either be dead or in some long-term mental health care unit. Although ECT is coming into favor again as a treatment for severe depression, as you will read in this chapter, the treatment still has a long way to go in order to overcome a bad reputation. It is my goal to help people weed through the myths, controversies and stigmas in order to make the right choice based on their own decision, after seeing the facts more clearly.

As a courageous survivor and advocate of ECT (electroconvulsive or shock therapy), I am often asked to speak to people suffering with depression and their family members about this treatment. Many have the exact same questions that I had when I was first asked to consider ECT as a treatment intervention for my clinical depression back in 1990.

Is it painful?

What if I awake during the procedure?

Does it hinder my intelligence?

Will it alter my personality?

In 20 years I have had over 50 successful ECT treatments during four major bouts with clinical depression. The treatment not only gave me back the desire to live, but the ability to thrive in my personal and professional lives. ECT has become my "ladder out of the depression pit" for which I am most grateful.

It is still unclear why ECT helps patients with severe depression. Some feel that the electrical shock that induces a seizure somehow stimulates the brain's neurons and reconfigures chemicals in the limbic system that regulate and balance our emotions. Some say the seizure alters the body's hormonal system to relieve depression. I say that the electric shock creates just enough force to reattach the neurotransmitters in the brain that somehow unattached and caused the depression. Like putting Humpty-Dumpty back together again. Regardless of how it works and why it works – it is my treatment of choice. And today, an estimated one million people worldwide receive ECT every year.

The thought of having one's head "zapped" with electricity can be very intimidating. But as I often tell consumers – ECT does to the brain what a defibrillator does to the heart. Can you imagine talking someone out of getting their heart started once it stopped?

The Procedure

If you had a bird's eye view of the procedure, this is what you would typically observe from start to finish. The patient enters the room where the procedure is performed. The room is referred to as the "ECT Suite." The patient is asked to lay on a gurney. He/she is hooked up to an IV that contains anesthesia to promote sleep and a muscle relaxant to prevent body movement or convulsing when the electric current is administered. Blood pressure cuffs and pulse monitoring devices are put in place, as well as EKG leads to monitor the heart and EEG leads to monitor the brain. The patient begins drifting off to sleep. A bite-block is inserted in their mouth to prevent them from biting their tongue. An anesthesiologist places an oxygen mask over the patient's nose and mouth to ensure proper respiration. Electrodes are then placed on the patient's right temple and the parietal area on the head. The doctor adjusts the electric current to the lowest intensity and shortest duration needed. The doctor applies the electrical current by pressing a button on the end of one ECT "handle." There is a brief pulse stimulus delivered that lasts just one to two seconds. That pulse induces the seizure that will make the neurotransmitters of the brain once again connect. The patient's body remains relatively relaxed and still because of the muscle relaxant, but you will observe a slight twitching of the foot or toe during the induced seizure. This twitching is timed by a nurse in the room, to reveal the length of the seizure – approximately 30 seconds. The procedure is complete. From start to finish the entire procedure lasts about seven minutes. The patient is unhooked from all equipment and begins to awake. The treatments are delivered in "courses" of 6 to 12 treatments administered two or three times a week. Some patients continue the ECT in what are called "maintenance treatments," and many will continue drug therapy as well as talk therapy.

The Success Rate

The success rate, according to the American Psychiatric Association is 80 percent. This is considerably higher than the rate of most anti-depressants which have a 45 to 50 percent success rate. And the effects of the ECT are generally felt as early as the third or fourth treatment, whereas medications can take as long as six weeks to take effect. There is however a general lack of awareness about the success rate because many who have benefited from ECT are reluctant to promote it for fear of rejection or criticism. This point is discussed further in this chapter.

The History

The procedure is quite different today than it was in its infancy, so be sure when you research the facts, that you are looking at current information. ECT was first introduced in the 1930s and gained widespread use as a form of treatment in the 1940s and 1950s, for a long list of ailments. It was used to "control" troublesome patients and even used to try to "cure" homosexuality and truancy. When ECT was administered in the early years, the patient was kept awake, they were strapped down and their body would convulse violently. They often suffered broken bones and bruises. A long stream of electricity to both sides of the brain affected the patient's language and auditory memory, leaving patients mumbling and unable to recognize friends and family.

Making Your Decision

ECT is not the first treatment option provided. It is an option that is often suggested when a patient is significantly depressed and/or suicidal and when other common treatment measures have failed. Medications can serve as a very effective option, but there are some patients who see no effects, some that have adverse reactions and some that have side effects to medications. When medications do not provide relief, ECT is a viable, lifesaving option. In my case, medications were not having any effect and six weeks later, I was still suicidal; so ECT was administered. After the initial course of ECT I also engaged in talk therapy and received a variety of medications. The medication that had no effect on me prior to the ECT seemed to work better for me after the ECT treatments.

Just like medications, ECT has some side effects. Many people experience a headache immediately after treatment is administered. I felt that the headache was tolerable and lasted only about an hour or two after the treatment. I also experienced short-term memory loss from the treatments and that seems to be one of the biggest complaints from critics of this treatment option. For me, the memory loss was temporary and would fade like the headaches. For me, the memory loss was well worth ending the psychosis. I often ask consumers who are concerned over the controversy of memory loss, "Which would you rather live with – a crippling sadness and suicidal thoughts or some short-term memory loss that is most often transient?"

Most people are unaware that major advances have been made concerning ECT.

The use of anesthesia and muscle relaxers – The patient receives an IV drip with a muscle relaxant that prevents their body from convulsing and an anesthetic to ensure they stay asleep through the brief procedure.

The use of unilateral ECT – Electrodes are placed only on the non-dominant side of the patient's head to protect the side where language and auditory memory resides. Bi-lateral ECT is also used and some say it is more effective.

The use of brief pulse stimulus – This provides a rapid pulse of electricity instead of a steady stream; this minimizes cognitive difficulties as a result of treatment.

When making a life-changing decision, it is always helpful to hear about others who have gone through what you are considering. I found comfort in learning that valuable contributors to our society, like Mike Wallace, Kitty Dukakis, Dick Cavett and Carrie Fisher had undergone ECT and found it very successful in treating their depression.

The Stigma Effect

The National Alliance on Mental Illness (NAMI) conducted a recent survey to reveal gaps in Americans' understanding of major depression and treatment options. Over 500 people living with depression were polled. The majority of them (67 percent) use psychiatric medications as their primary treatment, compared to only one percent who uses ECT. Of the 67 percent who chose medications, approximately half of them felt the medications were not helping. Many claimed they stopped taking the medications due to adverse side-effects. Therefore, a staggering number of individuals who have abandoned their medications are still potentially struggling with depression yet have dismissed ECT as a viable alternative.

Even more distressing, the survey shows the treatment options that people living with depression have chosen over ECT include psychotherapy, prayer and spiritual practices, physical exercise, herbal or nutritional remedies, peer education and support, meditation or yoga, animal therapy, music and art therapy, massage therapy and other body work. While all of these options have value, it is discouraging to think that ECT is thought of as either a last resort or not considered at all.

So what causes the public to harbor such a negative view of the procedure and dismiss it before careful consideration? Thoughts, words, images... electricity to the body conjures up thoughts of the electric chair used for punishing the nastiest of criminals. Even the word "shock" carries a negative connotation reinforced by outdated images kept alive by Hollywood, from early ECT treatments and frightening images of patients grimacing in pain during a treatment. Say the words "shock therapy" to ten people and nine of them will respond with the movie title "One Flew Over the Cuckoo's Nest." The movie (made in 1975) won five academy awards, but left a wretched taste in our mouths about ECT. That movie as well as "The Snake Pit" (made in 1945) both depict the earlier developments of the treatment – not the modernized procedure that provides relief to countless patients every day. Unfortunately, they have left a deep impression on society that ECT is not only painful, barbaric and inhumane, but something to be ashamed of.

The fact is those images are far from the current reality. Like all medical treatments, time and science have brought major advancements to the treatment. When you think about the fact that surgeons used to put their hands in open wounds without wearing gloves, operated without sterilizing instruments or without using anesthetics, you realize how much more advanced modern medicine is now and that includes ECT.

As with any treatment for any illness, there is always controversy. I am a firm believer in asking the questions and weighing the options when making the best choice for you, **regardless of what anyone else thinks.** One of the biggest controversies concerning ECT is revealed in a question often heard when I advocate for the treatment:

How will people react to me if I use this treatment?

I can absolutely appreciate this question as it was the one I asked myself over and over when I was trying to make the decision. I worried that my colleagues would look down on me, that my boss wouldn't want to employ me anymore, that my children's friends wouldn't be allowed to play in my house. Again, this is why I do what I do now. I want people to see the results of the treatment through my own model. "The proof is in the pudding," as they say.

Controversial attitudes can get vicious as is seen by many chat rooms and blog postings on line. Judgmental comments are often angrily expressed by people who haven't undergone ECT. This is extremely distressing. Even if a person is unafraid of the treatment, they may decline because they are intimidated by the judgment and criticism of others. **I urge those who have had success to share their stories.** In this age of technology, it is very easy to share your positive experiences with others by a few taps on the keyboard. Don't be afraid. Take it upon yourself to openly share how ECT has helped you. Who knows? You may even save a life!

Together we can transform the face of ECT.

Will I Ever Be the Same Again?

CHAPTER 10
A Courageous Recovery Wellness Model

Years of interaction with those directly or indirectly affected by depression inspired me to create a basic tool to assist consumers in achieving wellness that is sustainable, or at the very least, a wellness that becomes a home base between depressive episodes. I call this tool the "Courageous Recovery Wellness Model," and it consists of three necessary attributes – each building on the one that precedes it. A visual of this model is shown on page 67.

The three attributes are awareness, acceptance and commitment. It is my experience that wellness is extremely difficult to achieve without all three of these attributes. I am certain that as you become more and more familiar with each attribute and take the steps that each one advises, you will enhance your ability to recover and return to wellness.

The wellness model is not just for consumers. It is a tool to aid the consumer's family members and loved ones, as well as their health care providers. The wellness model sheds light on the misunderstood and often judged diagnosis of depression, as well as a treatment that is extremely viable (ECT) and yet surrounded by stigma that tend to keep it locked in the closet so to speak. The wellness model will also help the network of people who are in place to support the consumer both during and between major episodes – family, friends, doctors, nurses, and anyone else who touches the life of the consumer.

After the visual of the model shown on page 67, I define each of the attributes briefly. Then, throughout the remainder of the book, I provide much more detail about how the model can aid a person.

Consumers (Chapter 11)
Loved ones (Chapter 12)
Health care providers (Chapter 13)

Will I Ever Be the Same Again?

A COURAGEOUS RECOVERY WELLNESS MODEL™

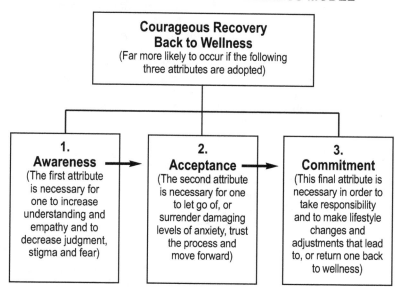

Awareness *(definition in Dictionary.com)*
1. Having knowledge; conscious; cognizant.
2. Being informed; alert; knowledgeable.

The antonym for awareness is oblivious. With lack of knowledge concerning depression, I was oblivious to what was behind the myriad of symptoms I experienced when I was first diagnosed with clinical depression. I was also filled with shame once I was given the diagnosis, and that shame increased the ferocity of the depression. Therefore, I feel awareness is the first step to wellness. Awareness is freeing. It helps the consumer to feel less derailed when depressive episodes come along, and it helps loved ones to not only understand the needs of the ill individual, but to avoid the tendency to become judgmental.

Acceptance *(definition in Dictionary.com)*
1. The act of taking or receiving something offered.
2. Favorable reception; approval; favor.
3. Belief in something; agreement.

The antonym for acceptance is rejection. Many people reject those who are depressed. Many who are clinically depressed reject the reality of the diagnosis or certain treatment options like ECT. It took four hospitalizations and more than 50 ECT treatments for me to fully accept clinical depression as the diagnosis I would contend with for the remainder of my life. Acceptance cannot occur without awareness, and that is why it is the second attribute of the wellness model. Acceptance is a foundation for trust to grow. Acceptance prevents us from fighting the process and staying stuck. It is essential for the consumer to be able to move forward towards a treatment plan and it helps loved ones to make necessary adjustments in support of the consumer.

Commitment *(definition in Dictionary.com)*
1. The act of engaging oneself.
2. A pledge or promise; obligation.
3. An agreement to do something.

The antonym for commitment is indifference. Indifference is the enemy of an action plan. When one is unaware of the facts and unable to accept a diagnosis or a particular treatment, there is no way they will be able to comply with a healthy new regimen let alone a treatment plan. During my hospital stay I constantly heard health care professionals including psychiatrists say "the consumer is non-compliant." Compliance is something someone else wants from us, where as commitment is a choice we are willing to make once we have gained awareness and acceptance. In other words, get a consumer to the point of commitment before expecting them to be compliant. Commitment means the consumer makes a conscious decision to grab a hold of wellness by making necessary lifestyle changes like diet and nutrition, medication, exercise, meditation or whatever routines will encourage wellness. Commitment to get better is very unlikely without awareness and acceptance and that is why it is the third and final step in the wellness model.

CHAPTER 11

Consumers and the Wellness Model

I have often thought that the word "consumer" was a strange choice to be used in describing someone suffering from depression. Society refers to those who seek medical attention for anything involving their *physical* well-being as a "patient." Why are those of us who seek medical attention involving our *mental* well-being called "the consumer"? Who in their right mind would want to consume depression? But there it is – the beginning of a road of obstacles and stigma and self-judgment and questions and lots of decisions, not to mention the anxiety and hopelessness that depression already carries. I would much rather consume a luxurious vacation!

I am a consumer and I connect with others like me through speaking engagements, radio and television interviews and at association meetings and conferences. There is comfort in numbers, and in the company of those with whom we can relate. So I applaud you for picking up this book and connecting with someone who understands what you are going through. Recovery comes to those who take steps – baby steps included.

In Chapter 10, I introduced the "Courageous Recovery Wellness Model." A visual of the *entire* model is shown on page 67. The remainder of this chapter guides you to apply each part of the model to your journey, with the intention of returning you to wellness.

1. **Awareness** (Necessary for one to increase understanding and empathy and to decrease judgment, stigma and fear)	Awareness is the first step to wellness. It opens our eyes and gives us a different perspective. As we become more aware we become less afraid. Fear stops us from moving forward. By becoming more knowledgeable, we reduce our levels of fear and remove the wall that blocks our forward progress.

There is a phrase, "you don't know what you don't know." Depression came as a complete surprise to me based on what I didn't know. In other words, if you have no knowledge about depression, nor know someone with depression and it suddenly comes knocking at your door, chances are you will be completely caught off guard and confused by the symptoms. But in this day and age, with television commercials advertising a variety of new anti-depressants daily, very few of us aren't at least somewhat aware of the meaning of depression. And according to the National Institute of Mental Health, 15 million Americans are diagnosed with depression annually, making it very likely that all of us know someone directly or indirectly who has dealt with depression, whether it's situational, clinical, manic, post-partum, or even seasonal affective disorder.

As I've discussed throughout the book, the causes of depression are varied – factors that contribute to depression include, genetics, biology, chemistry, hormones, environment, psychology and socio-economic.

In my case, I felt thrown for a loop when I encountered the symptoms of depression because as far as I knew at that time, there was no depression in my family history, I wasn't particular distressed by anything in life, and I wasn't going through menopause or any kind of grief or sadness. To the contrary, I felt I had the world by the strings and was very happy with most aspects of my life. For me, becoming aware of depression was like removing the skins of an onion, one at a time. Each symptom I encountered would send me to my doctor to eliminate yet another diagnosis until he finally exhausted all possibilities. Had I been more aware of depression and the symptoms, I would have found the illness less puzzling.

If you took the depression assessment offered in Chapter 8, you have an understanding of some of the symptoms associated with depression as they are asked in question form. Below, I include a list of symptoms put together by the National Institute of Mental Health. Keep in mind that the severity and frequency of symptoms and how long they last vary depending on the individual.

- Persistent sad, anxious or "empty" feelings
- Feelings of hopelessness and/or pessimism
- Irritability, restlessness, anxiety
- Feelings of guilt, worthlessness and/or helplessness
- Loss of interest in activities or hobbies once pleasurable, including sex

- Fatigue and decreased energy
- Difficulty concentrating, remembering details and making decisions
- Insomnia, waking up during the night, or excessive sleeping
- Overeating or appetite loss
- Thoughts of suicide or suicide attempts
- Persistent aches or pains, headaches, cramps or digestive problems that do not ease even with treatment

Even the most severe cases of depression are highly treatable, but it is important to remember that the earlier treatment begins, the more effective it is and the greater the likelihood that a recurrence of the depression can be prevented. A doctor or mental health professional will conduct a complete diagnostic evaluation as well as a family history. Once diagnosed, a person with depression can be treated with a number of methods. The most common treatment methods are medication and psychotherapy. For cases like mine, where medication and talk therapy did not alleviate the depression, ECT may be useful (for more information about ECT see Chapter 9).

Individuals who are in a depressed state are usually quick to judge themselves, yet slow to take action to help themselves. It can be extremely difficult to help yourself if you are severely depressed. In my case, anxiety clouded everything and left me literally standing by the window for hours obsessing over everything in life. It is important to realize that these *feelings are part of the depression* and do not reflect actual circumstances. Part of the Beast of depression is the way it completely blows situations out of proportion. Normal obstacles of the human journey can derail one in the midst of a severe episode, thus adding to the depression. Depression feeds obsession – obsession feeds depression until the Beast is so overwhelming that finding ways to escape the psychosis becomes a priority. *Treatment is critical.* As you become aware of your type of depression and you begin treatment that works for you, obsessive thinking will fade away.

To increase awareness about depression and to move towards recovery, it is vital that you stay connected with others – in other words, *don't alienate yourself.* Alienation feeds the Beast by doing a major disservice to your mind. We begin to feel like a misfit and we fool ourselves into believing that no one wants to be around us, that we should hide from society and that nothing will help us. Instead, educate yourself as you would with any other illness, through research, conversations, questions, and engage in positive direct personal contact with people affected by clinical depression. There are so many wonderful organizations where people can go to learn more about their illness, to meet others with whom they can relate, and where they get support from people who understand. (See the Resource section for some suggestions.)

To aid in your awareness about depression, I offer the following food for thought:

- If you are clinically depressed, you have the same rights as everyone else – the right to engage in meaningful work, access to healthcare, positive relationships, decent affordable housing, sufficient public education, and acceptance by your family and peers.

- If you are clinically depressed, you can recover and live a productive life – holding a job, going back to school, having close personal relationships, and reaching your full potential.
- If you are clinically depressed, you have the right to choose your treatment and make decisions for yourself. In other words, you are still in control of your own life.
- If you are clinically depressed, you are just as much a productive member of society as someone without the diagnosis – it helped me to know that valuable contributors to society, like Abraham Lincoln, Winston Churchill and Mike Wallace, all had depression.

Beware of things that hinder awareness. Of the 15 million Americans diagnosed with depression annually, only eight million seek help. That's only a little more than half. Despite more openness about these disorders, stigma is still the major obstacle to awareness and understanding of this illness. Stigma concerning depression have consumers conclude that they are failures or they are weak or they have little to be proud of. It is disheartening to believe that others will be afraid of us, think less of us, or shun us because of our diagnosis.

According to an article by NAMI (National Alliance on Mental Illness) regarding a survey on the awareness of depression, "despite better awareness of major depression and its consequences, the survey indicates that stigma still persists: nearly 20 percent of the public view major depression as a sign of personal weakness, and 23 percent would be embarrassed to tell others if a family member were diagnosed with the illness. Fifty-five percent of Americans would be uncomfortable dating a person diagnosed with depression."

Undoubtedly stigma and use of labels can hinder one's ability to acknowledge the illness. But what causes the stigma and labels? Ignorance and lack of understanding, preconceived notions, fear and folklore as well as media's portrayal of the mentally ill, all contribute. Other people's skewed opinions and use of labels contribute to a lack of awareness, often by shutting us down and leaving us less likely to glean the information we need to get better. And believe it or not, people with the most intelligence among us can make statements with the least intelligence. Not long ago a highly-educated individual, someone whom I respected as a mentor, really let me down when she looked into my eyes and said, "You don't have depression dear, and you don't need treatment." What nerve! Would she say that sort of thing to someone with a physical illness? I can't imagine her saying "You don't have multiple sclerosis dear, and you don't need treatment." But it just goes to show how quickly people are to discount depression and make it something it is not – a weakness, a flaw in character or a pity party.

Other people's twisted opinions can be detrimental to our well being. Unfavorable or unsupportive attitudes toward one's illness is discrimination. Discrimination against people with depression violates their basic human rights. Despite the provisions of the Americans with Disabilities Act and other civil rights laws, people with mental illnesses experience discrimination in the workplace, education, housing, health care and at home. Most importantly, discrimination against people with depression keeps them from seeking help since it causes fear of rejection.

2. Acceptance (Necessary for one to let go of, or surrender damaging levels of anxiety, trust the process and move forward)

Acceptance is the second step to wellness. It opens our hearts and allows us to love ourselves unconditionally regardless of labels and opinions of others. Judgment stops us from moving forward. By accepting who we are and what we have, we are more inclined to trust those who have our best interest in mind.

No one wants to hear that they have been diagnosed with a life-long illness let alone a psychiatric illness. It took 10 years, 4 major hospitalizations, which amounted to nearly 100 days away from my family, and close to 50 shock treatments for me to accept clinical depression as a diagnosis I would have to contend with for the remainder of my life. I finally came to realize that it wasn't my fault I had this illness. I didn't cause it, nor was it a punishment. It was a biological predisposition passed on to me from generations before me. A cousin once said to me, "Don't you remember grandmom staying in bed for days at a time?" And I remember thinking, "Grandmom had 12 kids – who wouldn't want to stay in bed having 12 kids to deal with!" But the more I spoke with family members, the more I realized depression was a common theme in my extended family and this fact alone helped me to begin to accept my illness.

Denial is the enemy of acceptance. Denial prevents you from taking necessary steps to get better. Would you deny you had cancer if you were given that diagnosis? Denial only serves to prolong the illness and increase its ferocity. The same goes for treatment. There are some that will never say "yes" to certain treatments because of stigma and a lack of understanding or even fear of rejection from others who oppose certain treatments. Would you deny treatment that could make you well again? And if certain treatments didn't work for you, would you simply give up or would you go to the ends of the earth to find the thing that could save your life?

To accept my illness, I did research. The more I learned the more I could accept my diagnosis. The final tipping point into acceptance was when I attended a New Jersey State Conference hosted by NAMI (National Alliance on Mental Illness). In a loving non-judgmental atmosphere, I was surrounded by people who talked openly about their depression. They embraced their illnesses and allowed me to finally accept mine, and I have stayed in recovery since that time. I have spoken to countless others who have expressed similar experiences – that once they were able to accept their diagnosis and let go of all the negative connotations and shame that surround the illness, they were able to reach a point of recovery.

The timeframe to accept a diagnosis is not cut in stone. Some people may accept their diagnosis very quickly while others take years to accept it. Unfortunately, there will be some that never accept their diagnosis. And as I already mentioned, the same goes for treatment. Some will never give into certain treatments that could be their "silver bullet," like ECT was for me. I am often asked by the families or loved ones of a consumer to help them accept the idea of ECT when nothing else has worked for them. I put a different face on the treatment that was once considered barbaric or painful by so many. As one who has had so many ECT treatments with such a positive outcome, I am able to give consumers a completely different perspective. This helps them to accept the idea of undergoing the procedure.

Many times those with clinical depression will blame something or someone in their lives for their illness. I've heard consumers say the following things:

My parent's divorce caused me so much pain when I was young.

My siblings were treated so much better than I.

I was bullied in school and I guess I just can't get over it.

I believe this type of thinking hinders our ability to accept our illness. It just displaces anger we may have associated with the diagnosis. No one should be blamed for your clinical depression. Not you, not your parents, not your spouse, kids or neighbors. It is an illness that can be caused by a variety of elements (as was mentioned in Chapter 8). Anger, blame and fighting the diagnosis only serves to keep you stuck and that is when anxiety has a chance to take root and grow like a weed. Letting go of anger, blame, guilt or disappointment will help you to reduce anxiety levels and move forward. I believe when you surrender and let go, you are officially employing the help of your higher power to put the wheels in motion. Let's say providence takes over and things begin to fall in place.

When I accepted my diagnosis, I mean *fully* accepted my diagnosis, providence took over and provided a whole new mission for me. Having already been in the public eye as a professional trainer, I suddenly realized I could use my ability to speak to large crowds in a different way. That's when I dedicated my life to helping others to recognize that clinical depression doesn't define a person, it is only a part of that person, and that ECT is a viable treatment option not to be feared.

Once you embrace your diagnosis, miracles happen.

3. Commitment
(Necessary in order to take responsibility and to make lifestyle changes and adjustments that lead to, or return one back to wellness)

Commitment is the third and final step to wellness. It opens our minds to possibilities and allows us to take control of our lives. It gives us a target to aim for with a blueprint to get there. Lack of planning keeps us stuck. By committing to wellness, we are more inclined to stay the course as well as create habits we can return to in the event of a medical relapse.

Whenever one is faced with a chronic illness, lifestyle changes are essential. Think back to a time when you or a loved one had to make lifestyle changes because of a chronic illness. What was the illness? What were the lifestyle changes? Those with psychiatric diagnosis must also make lifestyle changes to remain in recovery.

Lifestyle changes are not temporary. Adherence is crucial when committing to wellness. For instance, *it is very unfortunate, yet very common for those who do well on medications and get into recovery to then go off their medications and land up in a relapse.* Medication is one of the most common types of treatment for those with depressive illness. Even though I was medication-resistant prior to the ECT, medications helped to stabilize me after the ECT; and I am still on medication today. This third attribute of the wellness model is essential for those on medication. Please remember this important fact – when one commits to wellness, they commit to stay on medication for life. You wouldn't expect someone with heart disease to drop their medications just because they are feeling better. The following lifestyle changes helped me and I suggest them to the consumers I meet:

Commit to your medication – As I mentioned before, no matter how good I feel, I will never stop taking my medications because I made a commitment to my wellness. I often tell consumers who are thinking about going off their medications because they are feeling better, to consider the other lives that could potentially be affected if they stop their medications and go into a relapse. How will that affect your spouse? Your children? Or any of your other loved ones? How about your job – how would dropping your medication affect those you work with? Or those who depend on you? Is going off your medication worth risking those things? Remember, you wouldn't ask your loved one to go off a blood pressure medication if it was making them well. Commit to taking your medication for life.

Commit to your therapy – This is another treatment that works extremely well for me. Depending on where I am in recovery, I may go frequently or less frequently, but the point is, I commit to continuing regularly. Psychotherapy (also known as "talk therapy") involves talking with a trained professional. A therapist knows you, your situation, your history with depression and he or she is your ally. A therapist also has a keen eye for seeing signs of relapse even when we don't. Commit to therapy and keep your allies close.

Commit to protecting your sleep – One of the worst symptoms of my depression was insomnia because the lack of sleep fed my anxiety and contributed to my aches and pains. I need between seven and eight hours of sleep per night. When something comes up that doesn't allow me to get my full seven to eight hours, I am diligent about making up the sleep as soon as I can. I also avoid situations where I know I will jeopardize my much needed sleep. With every illness there are certain sacrifices that need to be made. To me, nothing is more important than staying in wellness; therefore, I commit to protecting my sleep.

Commit to daily exercise – We have all heard how great endorphins are for our well-being. A hearty morning walk can give us the boost of endorphins we need to feel good all day. The word "exercise" usually conjures up grumbles from most people, but I have found, I feel far better on the days I exercise than on the days I don't. Walking 20 – 30 minutes per day is an exercise that almost everyone can incorporate into their life. Whether you do it on a treadmill, in your neighborhood, in a local park, at a school track, just make sure you do it! Did you know your local mall is a great place to walk when the weather outside is unpleasant? Malls usually open at least two hours prior to the stores within them. Go to your local mall early in the morning, and you'll see many people with sneakers actually doing laps throughout the mall. It's indoor, it's free and it's a great way to get your exercise while you window shop. If you don't want to walk alone, get a walking partner. There are probably other people in your very own neighborhood that would love to have someone walk with them. One of my best friends met her walking partner at a yoga class. They found out they were neighbors and made a pact to walk together every weekday morning from 5:30 to 6:15 am. That was over three years ago. They both agree that they couldn't do it without the other, so they rely on each other to get out and hit the pavement.

If you are not crazy over high-impact exercise, swimming is a wonderful alternative. If you want to swim year round but you can't find a local gym with a pool, try a hotel in your area. Many hotels will sell inexpensive memberships to the local community. My friend swims at a Sheraton in her community. She not only enjoys the exercise, she's met many friends.

Going to the gym is an excellent way to get your exercise. I hired a personal trainer at my local gym because our appointments held me accountable to show up. I use the treadmill and the weights. Exercise is also important to me because certain medications can cause weight gain. No matter which exercise you choose, make sure to commit to it for the sake of your wellness.

Commit to a nutritious diet – The American diet is sad to say the least. We usually look for something quick, which usually means something unhealthy. My commitment to wellness enabled me to overhaul my diet. There is no need to hire a nutrition expert – most changes are common sense. The following changes have helped me to stay in recovery:

- Foods low in calories – I began to eliminate high calorie foods mostly because the medications for depression sometimes cause weight gain.
- Foods low in sugar – I reduced my consumption of processed sugar since it adds weight and can make me hyper or anxious or moody.
- Foods low in caffeine – Caffeine interferes with my sleep and promotes anxiety.
- Foods high in protein – Lean red meats, green

leafy vegetables and other foods high in protein increase my energy level and strength without making me anxious.

- Foods high in serotonin – Low levels of serotonin are known to increase depression, so I make sure to choose foods that promote serotonin levels (fish, chicken, turkey, bananas, avocados, high fiber cereals and whole grain products).

In addition to those changes, I also monitor my alcohol consumption since it acts as a depressant. People are often confused about fatty foods thinking they should be reduced or eliminated. It is said that too little fat in a diet leaves us feeling unhappy since "good fat" releases endorphins. Monounsaturated fats that are found in some nuts, olives and fish oils are best. Make sure you discuss any dietary changes with your doctor, especially if you are taking medications.

Commit to prayer time or meditation time – Quieting the mind is renewing. It reduces anxiety, slows the heart rate and breathing, and it allows us to be in the moment and forget about the past or future. I am an advocate of both prayer and meditation and found that even in the most severe moments of my depression this sort of practice was a relief.

Commit to protecting your boundaries and saying "no" – I often tell consumers "You are a human being, not a human doing." Think about how you treat someone who is dealing with an illness. You probably don't push someone recovering from a stroke to engage in activities that would set them back. You have every right to make the decisions that are in your best interest.

Commit to journaling – I believe great healing comes from journaling and writing down my feelings. I often figure out answers to my greatest problems putting pen to paper. Journaling allows me to vent my feelings which alleviate many of the obsessive thoughts in my head. Journaling also allows me to see how far I've come and that is very empowering!

Commit to asking for help – My family is a pillar for me. My sisters and their families as well as my children and their families, are a guiding light in my recovery. When we are in the grips of depression we are often reluctant to call on the people who love us the most. We may be embarrassed, feel weak or feel like a burden. Just as we would be there for a family member who is ill, we must remember that those who love us are there for us. It may help to remember that people really do love to help. People feel special when we share our deepest thoughts with them. It means we trust them and love them enough to ask for their help. Remember the last time someone asked you for your help?

Commit to getting support – As I mentioned before, there is comfort in numbers. I love my NAMI family who understand and accept me for who I am and what I've been through. There are a number of fantastic mental health associations across the globe that are waiting to hear you, help you and provide you with endless information to aid in your recovery. (See the Resource section for more information.)

Commit to celebrating your accomplishments – Celebrate the small and large accomplishments you make on your recovery journey. The act of celebrating pumps us up and gives us the energy we need to replenish our spirit and keep going. Any consumer knows how difficult it can be to do the things that in the past came easy when you are in the grips of a severe depression. When you are able to return to the tasks you once did, celebration is well deserved. Here are some of the things I learned to celebrate when I was able to do them again:

- Attending to my personal hygiene needs
- Cooking a meal for my family
- Shopping for groceries on my own
- Balancing my checkbook
- Taking care of my children without assistance
- Going back to work
- Volunteering at my church to facilitate a women's group
- Completing a graduate program in adult education
- Authoring two books
- Advocating in the mental health field
- Running a successful business

It doesn't matter how big or small the accomplishment, celebration will motivate you to do more of it, while telling the universe that we value ourselves.

Commit to trying new ways to get into recovery – Many people who have had former success with medications find they reach a point where the medication no longer helps them. After working with their doctor, and trying all different medications, they may still come up empty and the depression worsens. Sadly, many give up and look no further. Be sure to open your mind to other options. ECT is a viable option that saved my life, and it could be the thing that saves yours if medication and other treatments don't help you. Keep in mind these other options for promoting your wellness:

- Electroconvulsive therapy – ECT or "shock therapy" (discussed further in Chapter 9)
- Acupuncture
- Prayer / spiritual practices
- Physical exercise
- Herbal or nutritional remedies
- Peer support
- Meditation or yoga
- Music / art therapy
- Massage therapy or other body work

Most important, never give up!

Will I Ever Be the Same Again?

CHAPTER 12
Loved Ones and the Wellness Model

When you live with, love or care for someone who is in the midst of a severe depression, you know what it means to walk a tightrope. You suddenly find yourself in a difficult situation that demands careful and diplomatic behavior and your whole world seems to veer off course. As your relationship with the depressed individual changes due to the illness, you may feel hurt, misled, resentful, sad, exhausted, worried and a whole lot of other emotions. The experiences of the consumer's loved ones are challenging and often overlooked, and that is why this section is dedicated to you with the hope that you can strike a delicate balance that honors the consumer, while protecting your well being. The fact is, friends and family are a key part of recovery for the consumer, and so the healthier you remain, the greater support they receive in return.

I walk the road of the consumer, but I also understand the challenges involved with being the loved one of a consumer. My son was also diagnosed with clinical depression. Therefore I've been able to see this illness from the "other side." In addition, I speak to the families, friends and caretakers of consumers through my business as well as through my affiliation with NAMI. I hear the concerns, the frustrations and the desperations, and thankfully, I also hear the joy and the miracles of breakthroughs and changes in the perspective of loved ones. There are countless resources available to aid loved ones (see the Resources section). For the purpose of this book, I provide basic information to make your journey a little easier.

In Chapter 10, I introduced the "Courageous Recovery Wellness Model." A visual of the *entire* model is shown on page 67. The remainder of this chapter guides you to apply each part of the model to enhance your journey as the caretaker of a consumer.

1. **Awareness** (Necessary for one to increase understanding and empathy and to decrease judgment, stigma and fear)	**For loved ones, awareness is also necessary to:** • Detect signs and symptoms for the consumer when they are unable. • Avoid judgment, assumptions and stigma that prevent the consumer from getting help. • Better understand the consumer's feelings and actions.

If you haven't already, I encourage you to read Chapter 8, so you will have a general understanding of clinical depression, as well as the signs and symptoms. Chapter 11 will help you understand what the consumer encounters with the illness and what this book suggests to help them recover. Sometimes a loved one senses a change in the consumer before the consumer themselves. This is especially true if the depressed individual is a child or an elderly person. The important thing is to recognize that depression is distinctly different from sadness. In a severely depressed individual, you may detect changes in:

- Sleep – they either need more than usual, or they are unable to sleep.
- Eating habits – they overeat or under eat and experience significant weight changes; up or down.
- Level of energy – they are exhausted and lack all motivation for things they formerly enjoyed.
- Enthusiasm – nothing seems to get them excited, not people, trips, financial windfalls, etc.
- Self care – personal hygiene or the way they dress no longer matters to them.
- Concentration – they forget things, can't make decisions and struggle to focus on conversations.
- Pace – they walk and talk slower, think and react slower.
- Mood – they are irritable, agitated, emotional, and anxious and may even lack complete affect.
- Self image – they may express feelings of self-loathing, guilt or worthlessness.
- Socializing – they withdraw, alienate, decline invitations and seem uninterested in interaction with others, even those closest to them – or they may cling to others out of fear and insecurity.
- Perception – they have a distorted view of reality, obsess over issues, seem paranoid or unreasonably frightened, fear abandonment, hallucinate and in extreme cases, contemplate suicide.

If you witness some of these changes in someone you love, you will want to suggest they see a professional as soon as possible. Helping someone with depression can be difficult. However, increased awareness can make a world of difference.

Awareness means taking the time to learn with an open mind. When you are very familiar with someone, and their daily routine, you have a point of reference with which to measure or compare their new behaviors. That can be a plus because it enables you to detect these changes easily. But it is difficult to relate to something with which you are unfamiliar, like an illness you have had little to no experience with. Think about it, if you have never lost a child to an untimely death, it is impossible for you to relate to the parents who have. If you have never had cancer, it is impossible for you to relate to one who has. And if you have never had clinical depression, it is impossible for you understand the thought process of one who does. All too often, consumers feel patronized, rejected and looked down upon because even those who are the closest to them make statements based on inaccurate assumptions. Awareness is essential to eliminate incorrect assumptions, judgments and stigma. In order to help you relate to the ill individual, I offer the following thoughts that I, as a consumer (as well as other consumers with whom I connect) often think during the toughest stages of the illness:

I don't want to feel like this, I am powerless.

Please don't tell me to snap out of it, I can't control how I feel.

The obsessive thoughts won't stop, no matter what I do.

I know you want to help me, but you don't understand!

I feel like I'm living in some parallel universe where I can see everything, but feel nothing.

I want to get excited to be with everyone, but there is a "disconnect" I can't explain.

I don't even know who I am anymore.

I'm not a hypochondriac, I'm not lazy, I'm not negative and I'm not looking for attention!

I want you to hold me, and I want you to go away.

I know I'm not easy to be around but, you have no idea how much I need you!

Even in this day and age, with all the information available to us regarding depression, there is still a staggering amount of stigma attached to the illness. Stigma is detrimental because it prevents your loved one from getting the care that can help them and possibly even save their life. Of the 15 million Americans diagnosed with depression annually, only about half seek help. If someone you know appears to be severely depressed, yet is reluctant to seek help, your encouragement is crucial. Major depression will not go away on its own. Treatment is necessary. (Chapter 11 discusses various treatment options available.) Awareness aids you, the loved one, to stay level-headed when the depressed person has an episode. You will be less likely to take things personally, to be bitter, to say something you'll regret or to give up on the person with the illness. It may help to keep these thoughts in mind:

> No one is to blame for the illness. Depression is an illness like any other that affects anyone at any age, at any time. You can't fix the depressed individual, although you can offer guidance, love and comfort. During the most severe episodes, it helps loved ones to remember it is the illness "talking," not the person with the illness; especially when the depressed individual is especially irritable or agitated, mistrusting and paranoid. No one chooses depression and it can't be turned on or off by will. Depression is not a punishment or an attitude, nor does it have a motive.

In addition, here are some tips that will hopefully strengthen you and stop you from giving up on the consumer in your life:

If he zones out on your conversation, don't take it personally – it is a result of the illness.

If she sighs constantly, don't take it personally – it is a result of the illness.

If she cries at the drop of a hat, don't take it personally – it is a result of the illness.

If he wants to stay in bed all day, don't take it personally – it is a result of the illness.

If he is ecstatic one day and miserable the next, don't take it personally – it is a result of the illness.

If she lashes out at you and says something hurtful, don't take it personally – it is a result of the illness.

If she won't come to bed at all, don't take it personally – it is a result of the illness.

If he won't eat the wonderful meal you made, don't take it personally – it is a result of the illness.

If she doesn't seem interested in your fantastic news, don't take it personally – it is a result of the illness.

If he doesn't want to go anywhere with you, don't take it personally – it is a result of the illness.

If she obsesses over unrealistic issues, don't take it personally – it is a result of the illness.

Always remember, you can be supportive while setting your own limits. (I provide ways for you to set limits and stay strong further in this chapter.)

2. **Acceptance** (Necessary for one to let go of, or surrender damaging levels of anxiety, trust the process and move forward)

For loved ones, acceptance is also necessary to:
- Maintain a relationship regardless of the consumer's ability to recover.
- Live harmoniously with the constant changes the illness can encompass.
- Be "okay" with the cards you are dealt, and live one day at a time.

Acceptance is a personal journey for the consumer, but no different for the loved one. The family member must be able to accept depression as an illness in order to be an effective helper to the consumer. The consumer has a keen sense for those who genuinely accept them and their illness from those who don't. It may pay to ask yourself this question:

If I don't accept his/her illness, how can I expect him/her to accept their own illness?

Why is this so important? When the consumer doesn't accept their illness, they are likely to deny themselves necessary treatment and therefore never recover. Or they are likely to blame themselves or someone else. If they accept their illness, but sense that you don't, they will be less likely to share their feelings with you and that can be dangerous, especially if they are having suicidal ideations. Understand that "agreement" and "acceptance" are different. You may not agree with everything about their diagnosis, their treatment plan and their lifestyle changes, but you need to accept them. You are entitled to your opinion, but they are entitled to your acceptance. They are still in charge of their life and their decisions and unless you are in their shoes, you can't relate to what they are going through.

Acceptance from the consumer translates as *"I accept that I am clinically depressed by no fault of my own or anyone else. I am not being punished nor am I punishing anyone else. I understand that my loved ones may not support my decisions or may not even accept that I have an illness. That is their choice. I choose to accept that I can't fix this by myself, and I am willing to find a treatment that helps me to recover and live a good life."*

Acceptance from you, the loved one translates as *"I accept that my (friend/relative/significant other) has clinical depression and that it is no one's fault. I accept that I can't fix it for them, but I am willing to be there and offer love and support. I understand that I may not agree with all of their decisions, but I accept that this is their journey; and I choose to support them. I also understand that while I accept their illness, they may never accept it nor recover from it, and that I have no control over the outcome of any of this. We will take one day at a time."*

People who are depressed have a long way to go before they can reach acceptance. Acceptance will help you to be patient. It will help you through the waiting period before your consumer's medication takes effect. It will help you if one medication after another fails them. Acceptance will help you remain hopeful if treatments that are foreign to you are discussed and advised. And finally, acceptance is essential for you as the loved one, if per-chance, the depressed individual in your life never recovers. This is a sad reality that some consumers face and just as sad for the loved one.

Your acceptance comes across to the consumer when you show empathy and patience, agree their feelings are real to them and treat them as an equal with dignity and respect. Lack of acceptance comes across to the consumer when you minimize their illness *(Come on, it's not that bad…things could always be worse…why can't you be more positive?)*; when you try to stop them from doing something they need to do (like begin treatment); when you make them feel like a failure because they haven't gotten better; when you cut them short when they talk about their illness (discounting their feelings); when you try to control them by forcing your opinion on them or when you turn your back on them completely.

Even though loved ones usually have the best of intentions, if they do not genuinely accept the diagnosis of the depressed individual, their words and actions may cause a depressed person to feel worse. Test your acceptance by answering the following statements. Put a check in front of the statement(s) you agree with whole heartedly.

❑ I know clinical depression is more than just sadness and temporary grief.

❑ I believe that clinical depression is a chemical imbalance.

❑ I want my loved one to see a professional instead of trying to fix this by himself/herself.

❑ I support the idea of my loved one taking medication for life if that is what they need.

❑ I support my loved one in exploring all treatments until they find the one that helps them the most.

❑ I do my best to be patient when my loved one is in a severe depression.

❑ I avoid making patronizing or judgmental statements.

❑ I act as a partner in getting my loved one to a state of recovery.

❏ I do not stop my loved one from trying new treatment measures if others fail.

❏ I treat the depressed individual as my equal even when they are in a state of crisis.

❏ My loved one knows that I am here for them no matter what happens.

❏ I understand that recovery is not always possible.

If you checked most of the items, pat yourself on the back. You have mastered acceptance. If you checked very few of the items, I recommend you increase awareness of the illness by doing research and asking questions. Awareness leads to acceptance.

One of the best ways to gain awareness is through direct contact with other consumers and their loved ones. There are plenty of organizations, like NAMI, that encourage that type of connection. (See the Resource section for more information.)

3. **Commitment** (Necessary in order to take responsibility and to make lifestyle changes and adjustments that lead to, or return one back to wellness)	**For loved ones, commitment is also necessary to:** • Help the consumer make lifestyle changes they can stick with. • Promote a strong partnership through the recovery process. • Act as a "hope holder."

Through a survey conducted by NAMI, the main challenges noted by caregivers were managing time effectively, taking care of their own health and finding time for themselves and making ends meet financially. The caretaker's commitment is two fold. They need to commit to stay strong and see to their own health needs, so they can help the consumer to commit to their recovery. I often think of the example we are given every time we hop on an airplane. The flight attendant explains the need for us, in the case of emergency, to put an oxygen mask on ourselves before aiding our child. We are of little use to anyone else if we don't take care of ourselves.

In Chapter 11, the consumer was provided a list of lifestyle changes that are essential to recovery from severe depression, and they were encouraged to adhere to the changes. I ask you as their loved one, to be their coach and cheer them on and hold them accountable. Many of the lifestyle changes will promote your health as well, so a partnership in commitment will benefit both of you. In addition to the list I provided consumers in Chapter 11, I offer the following lifestyle changes to you:

Commit to putting your health needs first – You can't help someone else if you don't help yourself first. As caregivers, we often put those we love before ourselves, especially if they are in crisis. I urge you to tend to your own health needs and don't let anything slip through the cracks. You have more pressure on you than the average human being, and the last thing you want to do is jeopardize your health and the health of your loved ones. Commit to taking care of your physical needs.

Commit to your emotional needs – It can be extremely draining to support and care for one who is clinically depressed. Quite often it is necessary for the loved one to enter into therapy to keep their stress level in check. Therapy is a wonderful way to drain off the excess stress that you accumulate by caring for a consumer as well as picking up useful tips from a professional. Consider engaging in therapy for your own emotional strength.

Commit to getting enough rest – You need as much rest as the one you care for. Lack of rest can lead to anxiety, physical ailments and depression. After giving so much of yourself be sure to rejuvenate and get the proper rest.

Commit to daily exercise – I provided the consumer with many easy suggestions for fitting in a daily exercise routine. You may want to join them or perhaps you have your own routine. Regardless, there is no doubt about the benefits exercise provides. No matter which exercise you choose, make sure to commit to it for your sake and the sake of your loved one.

Commit to a nutritious diet – Caretakers are often too busy and too tired to eat healthy. Many times, they prepare nutritious meals for the person with the illness and neglect their own needs. I can't emphasize enough, the importance of a nutritious diet. Make a commitment to eat regular, healthy meals. (See some of the suggestions in Chapter 11.)

Commit to prayer time or meditation time – Quieting the mind is renewing and essential for one who is constantly giving their energy to another. This practice reduces anxiety, slows the heart rate and breathing and allows us to be in the moment and forget about all of our obligations. I tend to believe these practices lead to a longer, stronger life and that will benefit you and the one you care for.

Commit to holding out hope for the consumer in your life – I use the term "hope holder" for the individual who instinctively knows that the consumer struggles to see hope for themselves. In my case, my sister Lexi was my "hope holder." When a clinically depressed individual relapses into depression, they always think it is the worst one ever. That, unfortunately, is part of the Beast. Each depression feels worse than the one before, even if it truly isn't worse. Depression robs us of the memory of how happy we are and how much we accomplish in between episodes. In my case, I received my master's degree and opened my own business in between depressions. A "hope holder" can remind the ill individual of these things. When I was sinking fast into a relapse and convinced I would never be the same again, Lexi held my hands and reminded me of my amazing ability to bounce back, and she helped me to take a mental inventory of all the things I had accomplished after my former episodes.

Commit to setting your limits – This can be extremely complicated for the loved one of a consumer, but it is extremely important. You can lose yourself in the illness of another. It is important to set your limits, take your private time and renew yourself. I suggest you have another person available who can "fill in" when you need some down time. Sometimes it is difficult to know what to say or do to protect your boundaries. *What if they call me at all times of the night? What if their paranoia prevents me from leaving the house or enjoying my own life? What if their illness interferes with my work and puts my job in jeopardy?* There is a wonderful book written especially for caretakers and loved ones of the consumer titled, "Talking to Depression," by Claudia J. Strauss which offers suggestions to set healthy limits. Therapy is also helpful. Just remember, your health must come first.

Commit to asking for their help – Many times, loved ones are afraid to ask the consumer for help. They feel the consumer is too fragile or too sick to lean on. The fact is everyone feels empowered when they are asked for help. We all want to feel needed. Consumers sometimes express a spike in recovery when someone they have depended on asks for their help in return (this of course depends on where they are in recovery). When you let down your guard and ask the consumer for their help or advice in your life, you convey a feeling of trust in them, and this is a strong pill to one who may constantly feel like a burden or a failure. Remember the last time someone you care about asked you for your help?

Commit to getting support – There are a number of fantastic mental health associations waiting to help not only the consumer but, you, the loved one. They offer support, advocacy, advice and so many tips to make your life easier. They bring in speakers with new ideas; they discuss new treatment options and there is a feeling of camaraderie amongst the guests and members. (See the Resource section for more information.) If you participate in association meetings, the consumer you care for is more inclined to do the same. I can tell you as a consumer, getting involved with NAMI was pivotal to my recovery.

Commit to making yourself happy regardless of the situation – In the case of a severely depressed consumer, I often hear loved ones say things like: *"I find it hard to have fun or feel happy when I know my (consumer) is so unhappy. I try so hard to enjoy myself, but I catch myself feeling guilty knowing they are in a constant state of despair. Sometimes I feel like I have no right to be happy while they are in such a bad state."* The best advice I can offer in this case is summed up in a quote that a friend shared with me – "Your living small benefits no one." When you enjoy your life regardless of the situation, when you allow yourself to be truly happy, you are healthier for everyone else. And no matter what the outward appearances suggest, deep down inside the consumer wants you to be happy.

Finally, congratulate yourself for the commitment of service you have made to the consumer in your life. The one who leans on you, who depends on you...the one that sometimes screams at you, zones out on you, backs away from you and then clings to you...whether they express it to you or not, appreciates you and all you do for them, more than you know.

CHAPTER 13
Health Care Providers and the Wellness Model

As a health care provider, the consumer depends on you more than you may know. You can make the difference between "full recovery" and "giving up" in the life of the consumer you treat. As a consumer advocate, I hear firsthand what consumers say about their experiences with those to whom they entrust their mental health and well being. Therefore, I dedicate this chapter to you.

From time to time throughout the history of my own illness, I have been blessed to be in the care of "angels" called health care providers. I share stories with my loved ones, with consumers and with doctors, nurses and other providers with whom I speak, of the times when these "angels" have done or said something that promoted my recovery when my chances seemed slim. I will be forever grateful.

There are also times when I've been in the care of health care providers who are less than compassionate and have made the road to recovery more difficult. Health care providers are integral to the recovery of the consumer, but they may lose sight of the consumer's perspective of depression as well as the needs of a consumer in the darkest days of depression. I will help you to gain the consumer's perspective by sharing my personal experience as well as the consumers with whom I connect every day. So get ready to learn what consumers need but are often unable to articulate in their time of need.

In Chapter 10, I introduced the "Courageous Recovery Wellness Model." A visual of the entire model is shown on page 67. This chapter will guide you to apply each part of the model to enhance your understanding of the consumer's journey.

1.
Awareness
(Necessary for one to increase understanding and empathy and to decrease judgment, stigma and fear)

How can you help the consumer achieve awareness?
- Put a face on the illness / give it a name.
- Let them know they are not alone and should not be ashamed of the illness nor their need for care.
- Provide information and resources and advocacy.
- Dispel myths for consumers and their loved ones.

In Chapter 11, this book spoke to the consumer with the intention of providing knowledge about depression through listing the signs and symptoms, the stigma, the various treatment options and more. As a heath care provider, you have learned much of this in your training. You are able to diagnose one with the illness through a battery of questions and tests and by ruling out other things. But in order to really understand the *journey* of the consumer, the health care provider needs to be in their shoes, and that's why I encourage you to read the former chapters if you haven't already done so.

Awareness is vital for a consumer to reach recovery. Awareness of the signs and symptoms, the causes, the treatment options, the high percentage of people living with the illness, the associations that can provide support and so much more. But most importantly, the consumer needs to be aware that recovery is not only a possibility, it is a probability. And that is where you come in. The consumer puts their trust in you. A high percentage of the consumers I speak with have said that their heath care providers never mentioned recovery to them. On the contrary, those with clinical depression interpret the messages they received from their providers as:

You will be struggling with this for the rest of your life.

There is very little hope of recovery.

Don't push yourself or try things that are out of your comfort zone because you can't handle them.

You should let go of many of the things you used to do.

You may not be able to go back to work.

Life will be demanding so lighten the load and accept that depression has you in its grips.

Obviously, those are not literal statements made by providers but with very little hope in the words or the attitude of the provider, that is what the consumer hears. I would caution you to steer clear of long-term prognoses that could limit the consumer's potential and inadvertently track them to fail. Remember, a diagnosis identifies the cause of an illness through evaluation, examination and laboratory data, while a prognosis predicts the outcome of an illness based on other patients' cases. However, an optimistic prognosis greatly enhances the consumer's chances of recovery.

Stigma is an important barrier to mental health treatment and recovery and a huge stumbling block to the consumer's awareness about clinical depression. I believe it is a health care provider's duty to help reduce stigma. The fact is stigma prevents many consumers from ever knocking on your door, so it is in your best interest to do your part to implement stigma-reducing initiatives.

According to the Archives of Psychiatric Nursing (Volume 23, Number 1, February, 2009) *"Underutilization of mental health services and early termination of mental health treatment are largely attributed to stigma. In 1999, the Surgeon General called for approaches to overcome stigma as a priority for the new millennium. In April 2002, President George W. Bush launched The New Freedom Commission on Mental Health, which strives to help individuals with mental disorders lead normal lives similar to individuals without mental disorders."*

In addition, many organizations have initiatives to reduce stigma surrounding mental illness. NAMI (National Alliance on Mental Illness) uses community education to increase mental health knowledge and reduce stigma through a program titled, *In Our Own Voice*. I was thrilled to learn about this campaign and became trained as an *In Our Own Voice* speaker. The program sends two consumers at a time into the public to share their experiences of living with mental illness and to relay the information to general and professional audiences.

Health care professionals are not immune to stigma just because they went to school and decided to treat consumers. Consumers often report hearing their own provider stereotyping and making jokes about those with mental disorders and depression. Even in the midst of a full-blown psychotic episode, patients retain their intelligence and remember what is said to them and how they are treated. I went to a new gynecologist who was going over my health history form. He asked me about all the medications listed, and when I told him they were for clinical depression, he actually stepped back and looked at me like I had two heads. The reaction was so drastic, that my knee jerk response was "Don't worry, you can't catch it!"

The stigma associated with ECT, in my opinion, is so harmful because it deprives severely depressed individuals the right to potential recovery. I had such tremendous success with ECT that years later when I had a severe relapse, I said to my psychiatrist (who was new to my case), that I wanted ECT. He shook his head as if I was drunk and said "Now who in their right mind would come in and ask for shock treatment?" I responded by saying, "Okay, you're fired!" This is not the attitude one should expect from their health care provider, but it is too often the case.

To help your consumer and their loved ones become more aware of depression, listen to the myths consumers and their loved ones often believe:

- If I have depression I should be able to take care of it myself.
- If I have depression, it is a sign of weakness – it's my fault.
- If I seek help for my depression, others will think I am "crazy."
- People diagnosed with a serious depression are always ill and out of touch with reality.

Those statements are common in the mind of the consumer and your ability to prepare a confident rationalization will help the consumer move toward acceptance.

2.
Acceptance
(Necessary for one to let go of, or surrender damaging levels of anxiety, trust the process and move forward)

How can you help the consumer achieve acceptance?
- Get to know them and their values, and treat them as a fully functioning individual (even during a severe episode).
- Relate their diagnosis to other types of illness and treatment plans.
- Discuss the positive possibilities and their ability to return to things they loved.

I don't have to tell you as a health care professional, the sad truth – that the percentage of consumers who will never accept their illness is still too large. You have probably seen this far too often in those you treat. Not to mention those you will never see because they refuse to accept treatment since they refuse to accept their illness. The goal of this book as well as my company's mission is to increase the percentage and get more consumers to accept their illness and get the necessary treatment so that they can recover and live a happy, productive life.

In this section I hope to open your eyes to the things that will help consumers accept their diagnoses so they can move toward committing to wellness. Consumers start to remove their self-built wall when they learn that clinical depression is like any other illness that needs treatment, so I encourage you to make that analogy for them. Just like a diabetic needs insulin, or an asthmatic needs an inhaler, one with depression needs medication, therapy or other treatment measures to get well. Consumers begin to accept their diagnoses when they learn they have the same rights as everyone else – the right to meaningful work, access to health care, positive relationships, decent affordable housing, education and acceptance by their family and peers. Consumers move further into acceptance as they learn they can recover and live productive lives, like holding a fulfilling job, going back to school and even taking on new challenges. They are encouraged when they hear about valuable contributors to society, who share the same diagnosis.

It took me a very long time to accept my illness, but as I mentioned in a former chapter, my tipping point towards acceptance was when I was introduced to NAMI (National Alliance on Mental Illness). I attended a state conference that changed my life. I was suddenly surrounded by others like me – consumers with clinical depression and other mental illnesses. They embraced their diagnosis and committed to treatment and went on about their lives – many, very successfully. Being part of a support network enables people with clinical depression to finally relax and surrender all their self doubt and anxiety and to be "okay" with their diagnosis.

A consumer is more apt to accept their diagnosis when they realize it doesn't define them. Just as a person with cancer is not defined by the disease, an individual with depressive disorder is much more than just that diagnosis. Providers should normalize the illness and the experience as much as possible for consumers. It is so important to let them know that they are not the only ones who have experienced this, and they should not be ashamed of their illness nor of their need for treatment.

And speaking of treatment, consumers who are medication resistance face another uphill battle with having to accept other alternatives that may be riddled with stigma like ECT. It was easier for me to understand the treatment than it was for me to accept the treatment because of my own misconceptions. I, like so many others, refused this option because I was afraid of what others would think about me. *What will my colleagues say? Will I lose my job? Will my friends ever look at me the same way? Will my children's playmates be denied access to my home by their parents?* Lucky for me, an angel in the form of a health care provider eased my mind and encouraged me to accept the treatment that saved my life.

Consumers are more apt to accept their illness when their health care provider feels like their ally instead of their judge. I have heard stories from some consumers about their providers that would make me cry. One woman's psychiatrist belittled her for self-medicating when she felt beyond hope. Instead of being the voice of compassion, he increased her already exaggerated level of guilt leaving her feeling far worse than before she met with him. Another particular man who finally decided to go for talk therapy, left mid-appointment when he realized his therapist was snoring. Drink some coffee or do whatever you have to, but never fall asleep on your consumer's watch.

One of the most common complaints I hear from consumers concerns the lack of bed-side manner belonging to various health care providers. Some will say "Why did he/she go into this line of work if he/she doesn't have an ounce of compassion?" Maybe the provider has a lot of compassion, but lacks the skill set to show it. In every profession, people can get lax in certain aspects of their job. Managing multiple priorities and trying to balance one's personal and professional life can over-shadow the things that need the most fine-tuning in our career. Corporate professionals spend countless dollars annually on improving their people skills to be the best for their clients as well as their employees. Although staying up-to-date on medical training, procedures and treatments is essential to your profession, please don't underestimate the value of your people skills. Compassion, dignity and respect in dealing with your consumers is crucial to their recovery. Test your "bed-side manner" by answering the following statements. Put a check in front of the statement(s) you feel average consumers would tell others about you.

The consumers would agree I:
- ❑ Make eye contact with them.
- ❑ Make them feel comfortable.
- ❑ Treat them with respect and dignity.
- ❑ Act professionally and ethically, but not superior to them.
- ❑ Talk to them on their level of understanding.
- ❑ Value them as productive members of society, and not victims.
- ❑ Listen attentively and don't make them feel rushed.
- ❑ Refrain from judgmental or patronizing comments or actions.
- ❑ Have a good idea of what they are like during recovery.
- ❑ Genuinely care about them.
- ❑ Have patience with their treatment.
- ❑ Make suggestions that they may not have considered.
- ❑ Am more dedicated to their recovery than I am to my consumer numbers.
- ❑ Believe in their ability to recover.
- ❑ Take interest in their personal life.
- ❑ Help them to see the potential in themselves.

❑ Share helpful information that goes beyond my call of duty.
❑ Made a good career decision in choosing my profession.

If you checked all of the items, applaud yourself. You are making an incredible difference in the lives of those you treat by going above and beyond. If you checked most of the items, pat yourself on the back. You are an asset to your profession and to consumers. If you checked about half of the items, you may want to beef up your people skills and ask for feedback from those who know you best. If you checked very few of the items, I recommend you determine your opportunities for growth and decide why you have difficulty with this necessary element of treatment.

For every negative story involving a consumer-provider relationship, there is a positive story that touches my heart. A consumer whose provider said "I see an active strong and positive role model in you and so do your loved ones," was the key to that individual's recovery. Another consumer told me how his therapist empowered him when she shared her own tragic journey of depression and recovery. He felt if she could do it, so could he.

I remember during one of my hospitalizations in a lockdown ward, I was sitting at a table with my head resting on my bent arm, just sighing over and over. My anxiety was suffocating me. A nurse asked me how I was doing and I could barely answer. Depression can steal your voice and leave you out of breath. The nurse being wise enough to recognize facial expressions and body language looked at me and said in a very matter of fact manner, "Not in this day and age should anyone feel like this. I will talk to your doctor and see what we can do to make you feel better, Carol." Within one hour I was on a new medication that relieved the anxiety. I thanked her for speaking up for me when I was unable to speak up for myself.

3. **Commitment** (Necessary in order to take responsibility and to make lifestyle changes and adjustments that lead to, or return one back to wellness)

How can you help consumers to achieve commitment?
- Recognize the difference between commitment and compliance.
- Empower them to make lifestyle changes that will foster recovery.
- Acknowledge their victories and encourage them to do the same.
- Teach them to recognize early symptoms that can signal a relapse.

During my hospitalizations, I overheard doctors and other health care providers talking about various consumers and calling them "non-compliant." The term can be construed as judgmental to one who is struggling to find a desire to live. Not to mention the fact that becoming compliant is impossible to one who has very little awareness about their illness, and has yet to accept their illness. Without awareness and acceptance, the consumer's chances of compliance are extremely slim.

Compliance is something that benefits someone else, whereas commitment is something we do for ourselves. That's why it is important for you as a health care provider to help the consumer get to commitment before you can expect for them to be compliant.

Will I Ever Be the Same Again?

How can you get the consumer to commit to wellness? By starting with step one – making them aware of their diagnosis, treatment options and potential to recover. Then move them to step two – helping them to accept their diagnosis by treating them with respect, dignity and by losing all judgment. Finally, commit to becoming their partner in this journey – by thoroughly discussing a treatment plan, patiently and genuinely acknowledging their fears, victories and the person they are on the other side of depression.

In Chapter 11, the consumer was provided a list of lifestyle changes that are essential to recovery from severe depression, and they were encouraged to adhere to those changes. I ask you, as their health care provider, to cheer them on and to become their partner in wellness. You can do this by considering the following commitments:

Commit to breaking stigma – There are countless organizations and associations that devote attention to combating stigma, changing policy, and decreasing prejudice and discrimination: *"In Our Own Voice"* (National Alliance on Mental Illness), *"Open the Doors"* (World Psychiatric Association), *"Depression is Real"* (a coalition of seven nonprofit organizations) to name just a few. The Substance Abuse and Mental Health Services Administration (SAMHSA) offers free training by teleconference designed to provide the most up-to-date research and information about programs within the United States and beyond that are working to reduce discrimination and increase social inclusion of persons with mental health problems. (See the Resource section for more information.)

Commit to discussing a wide scope of treatments – Some consumers feel that their provider only recommends treatments that the consumer is already aware of and certain treatments are rarely if ever brought up. In a study conducted by the Institute of Psychiatry, about half of the consumers surveyed reported that their providers never brought up ECT as a viable treatment option. They felt they were "inadequately informed about ECT."

Commit to optimizing your "bed-side manner" – One quick way to change your attitude and increase your compassion is to put yourself in the shoes of those you treat. How would you want to be treated in their condition? Or how would you want your loved one to be treated if they were your consumer? Revisit the "test your bed-side manner" assessment often and if necessary, hire a coach to help you enhance your people skills.

Commit to getting feedback from your consumer – To be a top-notch provider for the consumer you serve, feedback is necessary, yet often overlooked. The Mental Health Statistics Improvement Program (MHSIP) makes getting feedback incredibly easy and free. They provide surveys online that you can download and print for free to gain the consumer's perspective on the quality of service. You can easily obtain feedback from the consumer regarding their interaction with staff, their involvement in a treatment plan, their response to treatment and much more. A copy of this and other surveys can be found at www.mhsip.org/surveylink.htm.

Commit to providing your consumer with information outside your scope of work – As I mentioned my tipping point towards recovery was when I connected with National Alliance on Mental Illness. There are so many wonderful organizations that can fill in the gaps that health care professionals and treatments don't cover. Consumers find comfort in the fellowship of others who embrace their illness and share ideas for maintaining recovery. Be sure to recommend these types of organizations to those you treat.

Commit to seeing your consumer as a fully functioning individual – Remember the person you see in front of you during a severe episode is quite possibly the next President, Nobel Peace Prize winner, teacher, soldier, speaker, contractor, father or loving housewife. There is life outside of depression and nothing means more to the consumer than their health care provider's ability to "see" them as the person they were before depression took them in its grip.

Commit to being the voice of hope – As I said at the start of this chapter, the consumer depends on you more than you may know; and you can mean the difference between recovery and giving up to them. As a professional speaker, I bring hope to corporations in one of my businesses, and to consumers in my other business. People are drawn to the voice of hope like ducks are drawn to water. When we cheer people on and point out the potential we see in them, they are far more likely to see it in themselves. And I believe we were born to be the light for someone else. Be the cheerleader for your consumer. Celebrate their victories no matter how small and encourage them to do the same. But most of all – always, always talk about recovery.

As a consumer, we ask that you:

Accept, not reject us
Respect, not pity us
Admire, not fear us

On behalf of all consumers, I thank you for putting your heart into your work, for caring for your consumers and for taking the time to read this chapter.

Part III

THE NEXT CHAPTER,
8 YEARS LATER

Will I Ever Be the Same Again?

Thoughts from
Suzanne Fuller Camlin

Carol Kivler is a dear friend, inspiration and true blessing in my life. When she first shared her incredible story of being "brought to her knees" by depression and anxiety at the age of 40, it was hard for me to comprehend. Carol is highly educated, a successful businesswoman, poised and well spoken; head of her own company, tireless volunteer in the church and community and a very active participant in the lives of her children, grandchildren and sisters. It was hard to imagine that my caring and supportive friend had suffered from four separate bouts of debilitating depression in her life. How could she possibly have been in such a dark place? How could she have been hurting so deeply?

In reading *"Will I Ever Be the Same Again?"*, I learned intimate details of Carol's intensely personal and compelling journey of recovery and sustained mental wellness. Her willingness to share an honest portrayal of raw feelings, insecurity, doubt and hopelessness helped me become more in tune with depression, a subject dear to my heart. I thought of people I love, of friends and of coworkers who struggle with depression or anxiety. Some admitted they have had thoughts of suicide. Some even attempted suicide. I always wanted to help ease their suffering but sometimes, just wasn't sure how. At times I would fall short of patience and understanding, obvious keys to providing help to someone in crisis. My own frustrations and misinformation overshadowed a willingness to listen with non-judgmental ears. Reading this book - as well as Carol's subsequent books, *"Mental Health Recovery Boosters"* and *"The ABCs of Recovery from Mental Illness"* - provided me with valuable information and insight. Through her writings, Carol better equipped me to help those in my life suffering with either periodic or chronic depression. Bearing witness as she shares her incredible journey inspires me to never lose hope and also to help spread her powerful message of hope.

Over the years, I have come to realize the importance of Carol's mission to educate, enlighten and empower others to face their own struggles with courage and hope. I have come to realize just how extraordinary Carol Kivler truly is. She is a beacon of light, offering boundless hope for those suffering with depression and anxiety. I have also come to realize that we are neighbors not by coincidence or happenstance, but by divine intervention. Our paths were meant to cross.

Three years ago, Carol asked if I was interested in serving as a volunteer Board member for Courageous Recovery Inc., the non-profit foundation she established in January of 2015. I wasn't quite sure how I would help stamp out the stigma of mental illness, but I knew I wanted to be part of her mission to empower those who are suffering. Serving on the Board has given me a bird's-eye view of her unyielding commitment to others. By telling her story, by sharing her journey of recovery and sustained mental wellness, Carol has indeed put a face of hope on depression. Bearing witness to the people whose lives she touches continually inspires me. At times, it takes my breath away.

Recently, a decision was made to add a new chapter to this book to provide Carol's readers with an update on her work in the mental health field as well as inform them as to what's been happening with her personally and professionally. As you turn the pages of Conversations with Carol, you will also learn of an interesting development which brought Carol's advocacy in the mental health field into her professional world.

Carol Kivler: courageous survivor, trail blazer, successful businesswoman, loyal friend and woman of deep faith. She's also one amazing Mother and Grammy! Eight years later, Carol's message to you is Recovery is Sustainable!

Will I Ever Be the Same Again?

CHAPTER 14

A Conversation with Carol

Carol's readers and followers on social media are anxious to hear answers to many questions about how and what she has been doing over the past eight years. I had the opportunity to sit down with Carol and started with the question on everyone's mind.....the very question Carol asked herself back in 2010, as she wrote this book, *"Will I Ever Be The Same Again?"*

Well, Carol, are you the same again?
"Actually BETTER!" she replied. A deeply reflective Carol stated that *"no one is ever the same.... we all have new experiences and feelings, new circumstances, new challenges and successes. The good news is I am better than I have ever been!"* Carol looks at life differently now, cherishing each day. She recognizes she is more than her illness, declaring *"It is only part of me and the life I live. It does not define me."*

What does define Carol Kivler is a strong commitment to her family and to her Christian faith. Sharing time and experiences with her three children, their spouses and seven grandchildren as well as with her two sisters and their families is most precious to her. Family time is very important. Nuclear or extended family birthdays and vacations are planned well in advance to accommodate everyone's schedule. Personal triumphs are always celebrated and loving support and prayers abundantly given whenever needed. At the core of her existence is her faith. Indeed, it is what grounds Carol. Faith helped her recover and also sustains her recovery. *"God was with me in my darkest moments and highest peaks."* She embraces the lessons in the valleys to enhance the joys on the peaks. God continues to empower her, provide guidance and wisdom. Carol is keenly aware of the divine opportunities put before her which allow her not only to survive, but to thrive!

On a relational level, what can you share with your readers?

"When I wrote this book at age 59, I was no longer married to my husband of 31 years." Carol admits she's dated quite a bit in the last ten years and still remains friends with some of the men she dated. The most significant man in Carol's life remains her former husband, the father of their three children. A journey of forgiveness and of understanding is how she describes reconciling her feelings to come to this realization. Carol admits how much he has meant to her and still means to her. Over 31 years of marriage, they grew up together, raised three children and faced her *"darkest nights of the soul."* Through lots of prayer and meditation she concluded she will love him the rest of her life; she just cannot be married to him. *"He is who he is and I am who I am."*

Is mental illness a topic of conversation within your family?

"Before I wrote this book, I sat down with my three children. I shared my deep desire to write a book about my struggle with depression and anxiety as well as my experiences with Electroconvulsive Therapy (ECT). They were very supportive and told me if my story could help other families, it was my responsibility to write a book." Carol's entire family is open about mental illness which they treat like any other illness. Family members who are also challenged with depression or anxiety are fully supported and encouraged to share their feelings. There is no shame or stigma attached. Because the entire family is educated about the subject, they are aware of the warning signs and able to intervene right away. *"We are a family that believes in therapy, medication and confronting the illness head on."*

What do you like to do in your spare time?

"I enjoy reading and traveling, whether it be solo or with a traveling partner. Experiencing new sites, landscapes, cultures and food is a way to see what God has created around the world." Taking lots of pictures and purchasing a memento of each place traveled - be it a box of chocolates, a refrigerator magnet or Christmas ornament - are ways Carol holds her travel memories dear. Carol also enjoys gardening and her intimate outdoor patio area is filled with cheery green shrubbery and a wide variety of flowers. That tranquil atmosphere lends itself as the perfect place to start the day with her

daily journal writings, Bible readings and a healthful meal. It is no surprise to me she delights in gardening. Carol tends to soil with the same care and commitment that she shows to everyone who seeks her support and guidance. By sharing her personal journey out of the depths of depression, she cultivates hope and progress with kind words, compassion and encouragement. She focuses on the positive, pushing aside negative thoughts and fears that derail a harvest of mental well-being. Indeed, Carol is a master gardener for those suffering from depression and anxiety.

What's been happening in your professional life?
"Since 1994, I've been the President of Kivler Communications, a corporate training and executive coaching firm." An underlying desire to make a difference in the mental health field intensified in 2003 and Carol began speaking at medical schools, treatment centers and mental health conferences. *"Depression is an illness of hopelessness, an illness of isolation, and an illness of desperation. Since the individual is unable to feel hope, it is essential for healthcare professionals and family members to provide hope."* Carol recognized that these individuals were grasping for hope.....hope that their loved one would return to them and hope that their loved one would once again feel whole. Sharing her amazing journey from a person paralyzed with clinical depression to a compelling spokesperson for recovery instills hope. She truly believes that hope is the most essential medication in recovery. *"It has become*

abundantly clear that I have the God-given ability to empower others with a sense of hope. With this in mind, I believe with every fiber of my being that my responsibility and life purpose is to put the face of hope on depression."

Carol's bold proclamation - coupled with her steadfast commitment to share her story of hope and recovery - evolved, and in 2003 she founded Courageous Recovery, a small division within Kivler Communications. She continued traveling the country, presenting a wide variety of programs, both locally and nationally. By recounting a deeply personal and honestly lived experience of being *"brought to her knees"* by depression and anxiety at age 40, Carol educated, enlightened and empowered others to face their own struggles with hope and courage. Her steadfast commitment to stamp out the stigma of mental illness continues to this day. *"People with mental illness want to be viewed as courageous survivors - to be accepted, not rejected; respected, not pitied; and admired, not feared."*

So, how did Courageous Recovery, a small division of your company, flourish into a nonprofit?
"Through Courageous Recovery, I was invited to speak at nursing and medical schools, as well as at Ground Rounds in hospitals across the United States. I encouraged mental healthcare professionals to share messages of hope and possibility, instead of fear and limitation. I stressed the need for them to move away from consumer compliance and move toward patient

commitment. I recognized that our mental healthcare professionals needed to hear and see what we, who live with these illnesses, need so desperately from them."

This powerful message caught the attention of many healthcare professionals, resulting in widespread recognition of Carol as a very special mental health advocate. While the growing demand for her to speak across the country was very exciting, it posed an ironic dilemma: travel expenses were increasing so rapidly that she could no longer continue to absorb them. It then became clear that a much-needed solution was needed.

In July of 2014, Courageous Recovery was accredited as a 501(c)(3) non-profit organization, Courageous Recovery, Inc. (CRI). CRI's mission is to promote a mental wellness movement by advancing education, advocating nationally, and eliminating stigma surrounding mental illness. Serving as Founder and President, Carol put into place a volunteer Board of Trustees, largely comprised of healthcare professionals. Through donations, sponsorships and grants, CRI covers Carol's travel expenses, sending her across the United States, bringing her to places that need to hear her powerful message of hope. *"Each time a patient/consumer contacts me to hear, 'You can make it to the other side of this illness,' I know I am living my purpose. Each time I receive a comment from a mental healthcare professional telling me I've enhanced his or her understanding of what a patient goes through and needs, my heart soars with hope for other patients who will benefit. Each time I receive a call or note from a patient, who has read one of my books, listened to one of my interviews, or heard me speak, thanking me for putting the face of hope on their own 'Beast', I am validated that I am helping others."*

You say your worlds collided in 2013 with a single telephone call. Could you clarify what that means?
"In my Kivler Communications practice, I coach international executives for periods of six months. During one call, an executive opened up about his daughter's hospitalization for depression. Larry lived in Boston at the time and when I found out the hospital did not mention the National Alliance on Mental Illness (NAMI), I walked him through the national website and helped find a local NAMI chapter. Both Larry and his wife attended the NAMI's Family to Family program. At the end of our time together, Larry thanked me for introducing him and his wife to people who understood what they were going through. They no longer felt alone."

In a subsequent group of executives, Carol coached Howard from Australia. During the first call, he asked if he could speak about something personal. Like many executives, Howard had Googled Carol's name and took notice of her work in the mental health field. He had many questions about his own anxiety and shared his innermost feelings and fears with his trusted executive coach. Together, they found a virtual anxiety support group for him. Howard remarked that in less than thirty minutes, Carol had provided more hands-on strategies than both his psychiatrist and psychologist combined! At that moment, the personal mission of Carol Kivler - courageous survivor and mental health advocate - became uniquely intertwined with her professional role as an executive coach and motivational speaker.

I asked Carol to describe her initial reaction to the unanticipated merging of her professional work and life's passion. *"I looked up to God and said, now I understand!"* Her worlds had collided with a united purpose! Undeniably, the skies had opened, the stars aligned and a new constellation of opportunity was created. Carol agrees. *"I make my living through Kivler Communications. I make a difference through Courageous Recovery, Inc."*

Carol, there's no doubt you've touched the lives of countless people challenged with mental illness. Can you share a few of your most memorable interactions?

"The most memorable was when I was a keynote speaker at a hospital in Minnesota. Doctors, patients and the general public had been invited to hear my journey from the depths of depression. As I finished speaking, a woman approached me. She spoke very softly. She asked how I was able to be so comfortable sharing my very dark days when I thought of taking my life and the lives of my children. I told her it wasn't easy...that I used to shake, inside and out, and that it would take me hours to recover from the angst I felt. I let her know that the more I told my story, the easier it became. I asked why

she had asked me that question. She confided that she had had the same thoughts, but had not told a single person. I replied, well, you just told me. Now let the truth set you free."

Carol spoke of another special interaction she had while speaking at a nursing school at Seton Hall University. "I couldn't help but notice a young nurse in the back of the room. Throughout my entire speech, I saw tears streaming down her face. She was waiting for me as I came off the stage so I knew I had struck a chord. She told me she needed to apologize to her mother because she had always thought her mom was being a drama queen. She said, 'Today, Carol, you described everything my mom has always described her illness to be.' I told the young daughter to be sure to include a big hug when she validated her mom's feelings. Giving a big hug will let your mom know she is loved."

Carol shared another amazing conversation she had with a woman in 2017 when she was the keynote speaker at NAMI South Dakota. Two hours before her speech a woman approached her and said, "You're Carol Kivler. I want you to know my friend brought me here. I've struggled with depression for so long. I could not believe another woman has gone through what I am going through. She told me how happy she was that I spoke about my faith and the role it plays in my recovery. She asked if I believed people's paths cross for a reason. I told her, Oh, yes! I believe in divine appointments."

The woman went on to tell Carol that she had not planned on attending the NAMI conference, but something in her spirit moved her to come. She needed to meet Carol, face to face, and see her with her own eyes. Three months later Carol received a call from the woman. *"She told me that our encounter was the catalyst to her wellness and that she had been anxiety-free for three months. She told me I had changed her life."* How did this proclamation make Carol feel? *"Supernatural!"*

Let's talk about Electroconvulsive Therapy (ECT). When this treatment option was first presented to you, what was your initial reaction and what made you finally decide to have ECT?

"Like most people I was petrified. But I had been in lockdown for 24 days, resistant to intense therapy and a growing cocktail of medications. My family surrounded me with love, support and encouragement, yet I was not getting any better. I was at the end of my rope and had no desire to live. I was consumed with suicidal thoughts."

My eyes well up with tears each time I hear Carol recount this part of her incredible life's journey. The insurmountable and indescribable pain had caused her to believe that taking her own life was the only way out of the bottomless, dark hole she had descended into. "The Beast", as she named it. So powerful, so debilitating, so all encompassing. What about her beloved family? Surely her suicide would have devastated them. *"I couldn't think about anyone in my family. Not even myself."*

How long after the completion of your treatments was it before you felt better?

"My family noticed changes well before I did. They commented that I had more life in my face. I remember my son saying, you must be coming back to us mom, because you're putting words in the right order in a sentence."

Carol explained it was a gradual process accomplished with tremendous support from her family. She spoke lovingly of her parents, sisters Beverly and Alexis, and Aunt Bea, who all played an integral role in her recovery, assisting in every aspect of her existence. *"I felt like I had to learn how to live again. I needed training wheels. I could not ride the bike alone."* Carol described the day she was able to get out of bed and do a load of laundry as well as the first time she was able to make her children's lunches for school. A few weeks after treatment, she recalled being able to make an entire meal all by herself. Carol continued with talk therapy and a variety of medications. Little by little she blossomed and began a new way of living.

Have you experienced any negative long-term effects as a result of ECT?

"Yes, I did lose a percentage of my long- term memory." What percentage? Carol cannot say. Interestingly enough, it was her short-term memory that was affected while she was undergoing ECT treatments. She described it as *"non-existent."* It wasn't until a few months after the last treatment that Carol began to get

a grasp on her short- term memory. I couldn't help but ask her how she felt about losing some of her precious memories. *"I'm here to talk about it. I would have taken my life. It is a small price to pay, to still be alive. Family and friends agree."*

Would you undergo ECT again?

"Without a doubt", Carol responded, with no hesitation. *"I know it works for me. It does not work for everyone, but I am one of the fortunate ones."* Carol admits her answer would have been different, had she been asked seventeen years ago. *"My answer would have been no. Then, my goal was to get back to work. I was more concerned about getting back to work than with my memory loss."*

What would you say to someone considering Electroconvulsive Therapy?

"If nothing you are doing is working, you owe it to yourself to try ECT. There are no promises. It's a viable choice."

The science of Electroconvulsive Therapy has progressed rapidly since you wrote this book. What do you see as the most encouraging change?

"The stigma of ECT has changed in the last 8 years."

Naturally, our courageous survivor has been doing her part to educate others about this misunderstood treatment and to help stamp out its stigma. Carol told me of a divine encounter in her life: meeting Dr. Mary Rosedale from NYU Graduate Nursing Program back in 2011. Dr.

Rosedale introduced Carol to the American Psychiatric Nursing Association's Sub-Committee for ECT Nurses. This experience led her to become a consumer advisory board member of ISEN, the International Society for ECT and Neurostimulation. {ISEN: An international organization dedicated to promoting the safe, ethical and effective use of Electroconvulsive Therapy (ECT) and other brain stimulation therapies for the treatment of neuropsychiatric illness through education and research. https://www.isen-ect.org/}. In May of 2017, Carol spoke at the ISEN National Conference in San Diego. She told clinicians about ECT and how the treatment saved her life.

Carol has also been busy speaking to psychiatrists who deliver ECT. During a 2015 presentation in Toronto, Carol introduced the idea of inviting loved ones of the patient into the ECT suite, similar to inviting fathers into a birthing room. By doing so, doctors would help alleviate their patient's fears while the patient's loved ones gained valuable information and insight into this misunderstood treatment. *"The following week, a number of doctors gave it a try then wrote to thank me for changing their patients' experience and for helping adjust their practices to be more patient-centered."*

As an advisory board member of ISEN you have a lot of interaction with ECT nurses. What changes have they seen?

"A nurse friend and I were just discussing some of the advances since my treatments some years ago. An important advance is family members have become more

involved in treatment planning. There are also more options to lessen side effects such as memory loss. ECT treatments are now tailored to each patient's response as well as the side effects they experience. In addition, monitoring of results has become more routine."

What do you think your life would be like now, had you not had ECT?
"I would not be alive to answer the question."

What are some ways you sustain your mental wellness?
"Whenever I feel a heaviness starting to stir, I go in for a talk therapy tune up." Carol is keenly aware of early warning signs - sleeplessness, disturbed sleep, racing thoughts and convoluted perceptions – and takes immediate action by contacting her therapist. Daily anti-depressant medication and an exercise program are also keys to her sustained recovery. Trips to the gym three to five times a week are supplemented with walks around her community, a healthy diet and positive attitude.

Another way Carol sustains mental wellness is through journaling, which she's done since her last hospitalization in 1999. Each morning, she writes either a letter to God about what she is feeling or a letter from God, outlining what the Holy Spirit is saying to her. Included is a separate list of five things she is grateful for. Forty-five minutes to an hour is set aside to read daily devotionals and Bible scripture. *"It grounds me and sets me up for a positive and impactful day."*

Weather permitting, her devotional time is spent outside on her patio, with nature. *"It's my being time, not my doing time. I fill myself, my spirit with God's peace and mercy."* Seven days a week, three hundred and sixty-five days a year, her day begins this way.

I asked Carol about her amazing ability to maintain this highly structured morning routine. I was surprised to learn she does not view it as routine or regimen. While it did not come naturally and took years of practice, Carol recognizes the tremendous benefit. *"In quieting my mind, I am in the moment."* Carol admits there are times she would like to skip her "being" time, but she never does. *"I know the importance of learning to be."*

Can you share a few general tips for sustaining mental wellness?

"I like to speak of the three "D"s: Desire, Drive and Discipline.

DESIRE: This is your attitude. You have to believe you can get better.

DRIVE: This is your personal motivation.

DISCIPLINE: You must be willing to do what you have to do. You must follow through with what needs to be done."

You've received numerous awards and honors for your advocacy and philanthropy in the mental health field. How does this make you feel?

"I'm honored and humbled. Twenty-six years ago when I was diagnosed with major depressive disorder and

generalized anxiety disorder I could never have imagined the impact those illnesses would have on me, my family, and the many audiences that have heard and learned from my journey."

I have had the privilege of attending several award ceremonies honoring Carol. I asked her to share remembrances from a few, in particular:

The College of New Jersey's 2017 Alumni Leadership Humanitarian Award

In presenting their Leadership Humanitarian Award, the College of New Jersey recognizes an alumnus or alumna who has shown exceptional public-spiritedness or concern for human welfare through philanthropic activities. Of all the nominees submitted for 2017 consideration, Carol was unanimously selected as the year's recipient! In her acceptance speech, Carol praised her compassionate mother, whose steadfast commitment and passion to help others inspired her to do the same. *"This Humanitarian Award is dedicated to my mother, Dorothy Gennello Bystrzycki. My beloved mother was my role model for reaching out and helping others who needed a lifting hand. As a child I watched her give rides, pick up groceries for shut-ins, or drop off a home cooked meal to a sick family member, friend or neighbor. My mother engrained in her three daughters by her example......'We are here on earth to lend a helping hand, lighten another's burden, or share a message of hope.' Thank you for not only honoring me today, but for honoring my mother as well."*

New Jersey Institute for Nursing 2016 EPIC Award

The mission of the Institute for Nursing is to preserve the heritage, principles, values and practices of a healing profession through the support of scholarships, education and research. By developing, implementing and funding innovative programs and projects, the Institute is able to influence the practice of nursing professionals and to impact future care. In presenting their EPIC award (**E**xceptional **P**eople **I**mpacting the **C**ommunity) recipients are recognized and celebrated for their contributions to the nursing profession. Receiving this award was particularly satisfying as Carol holds a very special place in her heart for nurses. She has spoken at over 20 nursing schools and nursing conferences throughout New Jersey and the United States. Carol refers to nurses as her *"light holders in the darkness of depression."*

2015 Pillar Award, Mercer County, NJ Chapter of NAMI (National Alliance on Mental Illness)

Carol was selected to receive the organization's highest honor in recognition of her extraordinary 15-year contribution to NAMI Mercer's mission through volunteerism, leadership, advocacy and charitable giving. When told she would be receiving the 2015 Pillar Award, she remembers replying, *"What? I'm not even on the Board anymore!"* In true Kivler form, she is very grateful, but does not rest on her laurels. She forges ahead, knowing *"there is much more that needs to be done."*

How are you spreading your message of sustained recovery?

"I've written two additional books, 'Mental Health Recovery Boosters' and 'The ABCs of Recovery from Mental Illness'. Each Sunday for three years I blogged for Esperanza Magazine. In 2016 I was invited to be a part of a WebMD educational program and filmed a segment entitled 'Why Depression Keeps Coming Back: What You Can Do About It'. The direct link to view my segment is education.webmd.com/depression-that-comes-back."

In 2017, PsychU (University), an online resource for mental health providers, patients and caregivers, invited Carol to record four audio interviews. The four podcasts are entitled "How Nursing Professionals Can Bring Hope & Recovery to Individuals With Depression"; "The Other Side Of Psychosis: A Patient's Perspective"; "What I Really Need From My Mental Health Provider"; and "Patient Centered Communication In The Mental Health Field." They can be found on carolkivler.com, under the tab entitled, "IN THE NEWS." Also in 2017, Carol became a Stability Leader with The Stability Network. This is a coalition of people in the workforce who successfully live with mental health conditions and who speak out to change the narrative around mental health.

Look for Carol on Facebook, Twitter, Instagram, LinkedIn, Pinterest, YouTube, Google and Google+. Carol remains an active supporter of NAMI, speaking at conferences locally and across the country. The organization continues to hold a very special place in her heart. *"NAMI gave me my life back. NAMI allowed my children and grandchildren to go through life with a Mother and Grammy, in spite of mental illness."*

So what's next for Carol Kivler?

"I've been working on my next book, which will be titled 'Unwrapping the Gifts of Depression'. I've experienced and learned many things along my incredible journey. I have come to realize a great deal of good came out of all that darkness, most importantly, my life's purpose. I want to share the good, the positive, the 'gifts' so to speak, that I received along the way. In doing so, I hope to help my readers search for and identify the gifts they were given by their challenges with mental illness."

Will I Ever Be the Same Again?

Resources

Below are a variety of resources for information and help surrounding mental illness, depression and ECT.

American Association of Suicidology -
www.suicidology.org

American Foundation for Suicide Prevention -
www.afsp.org

American Psychiatric Association -
www.psych.org

American Psychological Association -
www.apa.org

Brain Stimulation Therapies – The National Institute of Mental Health
www.nimh.nih.gov/health/topics/brain-stimulation-therapies/brain-stimulation-therapies.shtml

Cleveland Clinic -
http://my.clevelandclinic.org/services/electroconvulsive_therapy/hic_electroconvulsive_therapy.aspx

Comprehensive listing of telephone hotlines and helplines -
psychcentral.com/lib/telephone-hotlines-and-help-lines

Depression and Bipolar Support Alliance (DBSA) -
www.dbsalliance.org

Esperanza – Hope to Cope with Anxiety and Depression -
www.hopetocope.com

Healthy Place for Your Mental Health -
www.healthyplace.com

Johns Hopkins Hospital -
www.hopkinsmedicine.org/psychiatry/specialty_areas/brain_stimulation/ect.html

Journal of ECT -
http://journals.lww.com/ectjournal/pages/default.aspx

Mayo Clinic -
http://.mayoclinic.com/health/electroconvulsive-therapy/MY00129/DSECTION=risks

Mental Health America (MHA) -
www.mentalhealthamerica.net

Mental Health First Aid 8 Hour Course -
www.mentalhealthfirstaid.org/cs

National Alliance on Mental Illness (NAMI) -
www.nami.org

National Association of Social Workers -
www.naswdc.org

National Suicide Prevention Lifeline -
1-800-273-8255 (1-800-273-TALK)

Psych Central -
www.psychcentral.com/lib/2006/an-overview-of-
electroconvulsive-therapy-ect

PsychU – Patients & Caregivers -
www.psychu.org/spotlight/patients-caregivers

**SAMHSA – Substance Abuse and Mental Health
Services Administration -**
www.samhsa.gov

The Stability Network -
www.thestabilitynetwork.org

WebMD – Mental Health Center
www.webmd.com/mental-health/default.htm

Follow Carol on Social Media:

Websites
www.carolkivler.com
www.courageousrecovery.org
www.carolkivlerspeaks.com

Facebook
www.facebook.com/CarolKivler

Twitter
www.twitter.com/CarolKivler

Google+
plus.google.com/+CarolKivler

Pinterest
http://pinterest.com/carolkivler/

Linked In
www.linkedin.com/in/carolkivler/

Amazon Author Page
www.amazon.com/Carol-A.-Kivler/e/B005GWWAT6/

You Tube
www.youtube.com/user/CarolKivler

About the Author

Nationally recognized professional speaker, author, international executive coach and corporate trainer, Carol Kivler is also a passionate advocate for mental health. A survivor of four bouts of treatment-resistant depression, she battled this devastating and debilitating mental illness with courage and faith to a full and sustained recovery.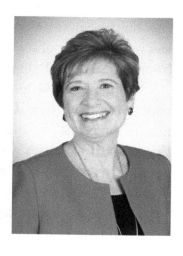

Carol is an ardent mental health advocate for consumers struggling with depression and mental illness. Through her four books, presentations and Courageous Recovery, Inc., her 501 (c) (3) non-profit organization, Carol works tirelessly to overcome stigma and misrepresentations that still surround those challenged by mental illnesses. She talks about her lived experience and shares strategies for maintaining sustained recovery and mental wellness. Her inspirational presentations resonate with mental and medical health professionals, consumers, their families and friends, inspiring compassion, understanding and hope.

Carol has received numerous awards and honors for her advocacy. Most recently, she was the recipient of The College of New Jersey 2017 Alumni Leadership Humanitarian Award, the 2016 New Jersey Institute for Nursing EPIC Award and the 2015 NAMI Mercer New Jersey PILLAR Award.

She is an active participant in the American Psychiatric Nurses Association Consumer Advisory Panel and past member of the International Society for ECT and Neurostimulation Patient Advisory Committee.

Carol received her bachelor's degree in business education from The College of New Jersey and her master's degree in human resource education from Fordham University. Carol has also received the Certified Speaking Professional designation from the National Speakers Association.

Carol is a popular keynote and workshop speaker at mental health conferences and events. She presents at hospitals, medical/nursing schools, continuing education programs, staff professional development, and CEU/CME courses. She is also in-demand at consumer conferences across the country.

Carol is a riveting, authentic and memorable speaker. Her high-energy and compelling presentations change thinking and inspire participants to reach beyond the myths and stigma surrounding mental illness.

Presentation Topics

Will I Ever Be the Same Again? A Recovery Story

The ABCs of Recovery from Mental Illness

Mental Health Recovery Boosters

Starting the Dialogue: Depression in the Workplace

Women and Depression: Awareness, Hope & Recovery

Demystifying ECT: A Patient's Perspective

Patient-Centered Communication
in the Mental Health Field

The Many Faces of Depression

For more information about Carol, or her company
and services, contact her at:
Carol A. Kivler, MS, CSP
33 Traditions Way, Suite 101
Lawrenceville, NJ 08648
609-882-8988
carol@carolkivler.com

Other Books by Carol A. Kivler

Blessings: My Journal of Gratitude
This interactive book provides a heartfelt way to preserve your recollections and move more deeply into self-reflection with your own blessings, to guide you with inspiring words, captivating watercolors, and different textures.

The ABCs of Recovery from Mental Illness
A handy pocket guide of 26 non-medical strategies that consumers can incorporate into their treatment plan to sustain wellness. Carol provides valuable information for consumers, their loved ones and health care providers.

Mental Health Recovery Boosters
A book of inspiration and reflection designed to move readers from mental illness to mental wellness. The 68 short but powerful essays stand alone with messages of encouragement and personal accountability.